Eat to beat your weight

Burn Fat, Restore Your Metabolism, and Extend Your Life.

By

Robert M. McNair

Table of Contents

Introduction

Sarah, a 35-year-old woman, struggled with her weight for years. She had tried countless diets and weight loss plans, but nothing had seemed to work. Feeling disheartened, she stumbled upon a book titled "Eat to beat your weight Cookbook" by renowned nutritionist Robert Mill McNair.

Intrigued, Sarah delved into the book's pages, absorbing the insightful guidance on mindful eating, balanced nutrition, and portion control. She decided to implement the principles into her daily life. Gradually, she shifted from fad diets to a sustainable and nourishing lifestyle.

As weeks passed, Sarah noticed changes she had never experienced before. Her energy levels soared, and she began to shed pounds steadily. The book's emphasis on nourishing the body instead of depriving it had a profound impact on her relationship with food. Sarah's cravings for unhealthy snacks waned, replaced by an appreciation for wholesome meals.

Her newfound discipline and joy in eating spread to other aspects of her life. She became more active, trying out new exercises and engaging in outdoor activities. Her confidence soared, and she radiated positivity wherever she went.

However, as Sarah's success became apparent, she faced unexpected challenges. Some friends doubted her transformation, while others felt insecure about their eating habits. She encountered skepticism and jealousy from those around her, making her weight loss journey emotionally taxing.

Despite the hurdles, Sarah remained focused and surrounded herself with supportive individuals. Over time, she reached her goal weight, and most importantly, she achieved a profound understanding of herself and her body. The "Eat to Conquer Dieting cookbook" book had not only transformed her body but also her entire perspective on health and well-being.

Welcome to the culinary journey that will revolutionize your approach to dieting and unlock the secrets to a healthier, happier you! "Eat to beat your weight" is not just another run-of-the-mill diet book; it's a groundbreaking manifesto that challenges traditional notions of restrictive eating and empowers you to savour food while achieving your wellness goals.

Say goodbye to bland salads and tedious calorie counting! In this book, we unveil a refreshing paradigm that encourages you to embrace the pleasures of eating, all while melting away those extra pounds. No more guilt-ridden dining experiences or feeling deprived of your favorite treats – it's time to nourish your body and soul.

Drawing on cutting-edge nutritional science and time-honored culinary wisdom, "Eat to beat your weight cookbook" introduces an innovative approach that celebrates the diversity of flavors and cuisines while optimizing your metabolism. Learn how to make mindful choices, indulge in delicious meals, and create a sustainable, lifelong relationship with food.

Our team of expert dieticians, chefs, and wellness experts has precisely crafted mouthwatering recipes, tailored meal plans, and practical tips to make your journey toward health and vitality enjoyable and effortless. Whether you're a seasoned foodie or a novice in the kitchen, this book is your key to unlocking a healthy and energized lifestyle.

Join the movement that has transformed the lives of countless individuals, shattering the dieting myths and embracing the joy of eating. Welcome to "Eat to beat your weight Book" your passport to a world of flavour, fitness, and fulfilment. Let's embark on this delectable adventure together and savor the rewards of a nourished, balanced, and unstoppable you!

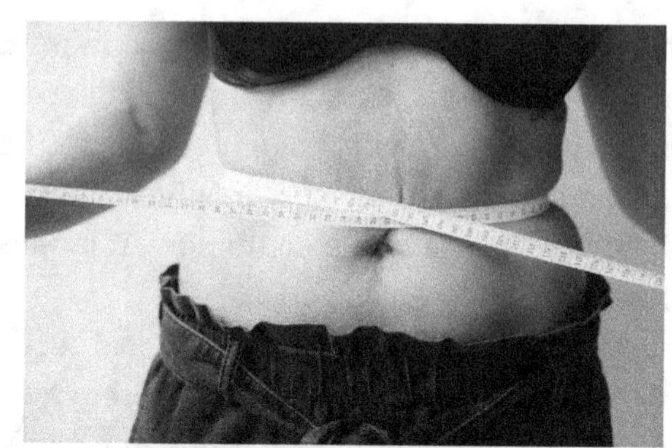

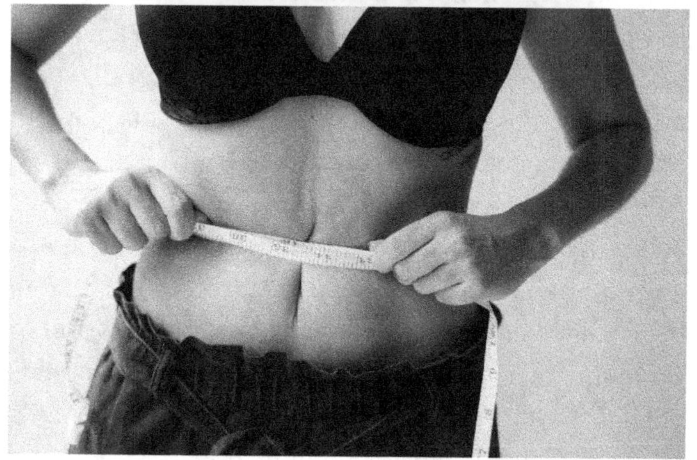

Chapter 1
Understanding the Relationship Between Food and Your Body

As we all know, Food is an essential part of human life because it gives us the nutrients, energy, and sustenance we need to survive and maintain good health. It is a broad subject with many facets, including its classification, definition, nutritional value, cultural significance, and the procedures used in its production, distribution, preparation, and consumption. The relationship between food and the human body is a complex and dynamic interplay that significantly impacts our overall health and well-being.

Our bodies receive the information and materials they require to function properly from the food we eat. In case we don't get the right information, our metabolic cycles persevere, and our prosperity declines.

Assuming we get a lot of food, or food that gives our bodies some unacceptable guidelines, we can become overweight, undernourished, and in danger for the improvement of sicknesses and conditions like diabetes, heart disease, and joint pain. So, what we eat is fundamental to our well-being. Science and workmanship manage the support of well-being and the avoidance, lightening, or fixing of illness. Food goes about as medication - to keep up with, forestall, and treat illness.

What does food do in our bodies?

The nutrients in food empower the cells in our bodies to carry out their vital roles. Nutrients are the dietary ingredients that are necessary for the growth, improvement, and maintenance of bodily functions. Fundamentals intend that if a supplement is absent, parts of capability and in this way human health decline.

At the point when nutrient consumption doesn't consistently meet the nutrient needs directed by the cell movement, the metabolic cycles are delayed or even stopped.

As such, nutrients give our bodies guidelines about how to work. In this sense, food should be visible as a source of "data" for the body.

Contemplating food in this manner provides us with a perspective on nourishment that goes past calories or grams, great food varieties, or terrible food sources. This view drives us to focus on food varieties we ought to have included as opposed to food varieties to reject.

Rather than review food as the foe, we shift focus over to food as a method for making Well-being and reducing illness by assisting the body with keeping up with capability.

The adage You are what you eat holds a lot of truth, as the food we consume directly influences our physical, mental, and emotional health. Proper nutrition is essential for maintaining a healthy body, preventing chronic diseases, supporting brain function, and sustaining energy levels.

What is a calorie?

Have you at any point looked hard and long at the names on the bottles, containers, and boxes of food in your kitchen? Then, at that point, you have likely seen their nutrition label. These labels give you the information you want to make healthy food decisions.

Energy for our body is provided by the food we eat. At the point when we digest food, our bodies use some energy immediately and store the remainder of the energy for some other time. Our bodies use energy for three primary things. These include digestion, physical activity, and other body capabilities. Ideally, we accept it as the need might arise. If we take in more energy than we want, our bodies will store the additional energy as fat. Assuming we take in less energy than we want, our bodies will get energy from stored fat. It's not a good idea to have either too much or too little energy. We experience, and ingest, them consistently. Yet, what's the significance here of eating a calorie?

A calorie is the amount of energy that is needed to raise the temperature of 1 gram of water by 1°C. That is, how much energy is expected to raise the temperature of one liter of water by one degree. Calories are regularly used to portray how much energy your body gets from what you eat and drink. Calories can likewise be use to depict how much energy your body needs to perform actual errands including Breathing, thinking, and keeping up with your heartbeat.

The amount of energy that food varieties give is typically kept in a large number of calories, or kilocalories (kcal). For example, one carrot generally furnishes you with 25,000 calories or 25 kcal. However, you normally burn 300,000 calories, or 300 kcal, while running on the treadmill for 30 minutes. In any case, since "kilocalories" is an awkward word to use, people frequently use the expression "calories" all things considered. For the reasons for this article, the normal term "calorie" will be used to depict kilocalories (kcal). Calories are used to portray the energy your body gets from food sources or consumed on different exercises.

Counting Calories

The word "Calorie" is gotten from the Latin word calor, which means "heat." The number of calories we concentrate from food relies upon which species we eat, how we set up our food, which microorganisms are in our stomach, and how much energy we use to process various food sources. Food marks contain the number of calories per serving. Be that as it may, how could this not be entirely set in stone? The response is shockingly straightforward: The food is burned. A sample of the food is put in a protected, oxygen-filled chamber that is encircled by water. This chamber is known as a bomb calorimeter. The sample is burned totally. The intensity from the consumption builds the temperature of the water, which is estimated and demonstrates the quantity of calories in the food. For instance, if the water temperature increases by 20 degrees, the food contains 20 calories. This strategy for measuring calories is called direct calorimetry.

Based on current research, calorie labels are simply expected to be an aid, not a precise estimation. The digestion of food in people differentiates and that can change the quantity of calories an individual gets from a specific food.

Generally, the average adult woman needs to consume around 2,000 calories per day, and the adult man around 2,500 to 3,000, While these numbers give a ballpark metric, calorie requirements differ definitely from one individual to another, How much energy your body needs changes in light of many variables, including movement level, age, level and that's just the beginning.

At the point when you eat a larger number of calories than you want, the body will change over that unused energy into muscle (transient capacity) or fat tissues (long haul stockpiling). This is an endurance component if you're not ready to eat enough, your body will take advantage of these stores to fuel itself. "The body indeed is this astounding machine," Consuming an excess of energy can prompt weight gain and medical conditions. A significant culprit in the U.S. where obesity affects over 93 million adults, is food sources with "empty calories." Soft drinks like soda are a good example. It gives no wholesome advantage and a ton of calories. In your diet, you need to get the most value for your money. You need food varieties that convey calories along with different supplements like nutrients, minerals, proteins, and fiber. At last, calories aren't the enemy. Many people hoping to lose weight get annoyed with the numbers; however, you should think about calories as far as your individualized energy needs.

How does your body use calories?

If you're asking why calories matter, it's critical to comprehend how your body uses them. It starts with what you eat. Food and refreshments are where your body gets the calories it needs to work. One of the three macronutrients, which together make up those calories:

Carbohydrates are also referred to as carbs, protein, and fat. During digestion, your body separates the food varieties you eat into more modest units. These subunits can either be used to construct your tissues or to give your body the energy it requires to meet its immediate needs. The amount of energy your body gets from the subunits relies upon where they come from:

- Carbs: 4 calories for each gram
- protein: 4 calories for each gram
- fat: 9 calories for each gram
- Alcohol: 7 calories for each gram

Your body uses the calories produced from using these supplements to control three primary processes, which are listed below.

1. Basic metabolism: Your body will use most calories to carry out fundamental functions, for example, giving energy to your mind, kidneys, lungs, heart, and Nervous system.

The amount of energy required to support these functions is referred to as your basal metabolic rate (BMR). This is at times referred to as Resting Metabolic Rate (RMR) because it refers to the calories your body exhausts in a resting state for getting through one day to the next. BMR (or RMR) makes up the biggest proportion of your total everyday energy prerequisites.

2. Digestion: Your body will use part of the calories you consume to help you digest and process the food sources you eat. This is known as the thermic impact of food (TEF), and it shifts given the food sources you eat. For example, protein requires somewhat more energy to be processed, while fat requires the least. Around 10% of the calories you get from dinner will be used to support the TEF.

3. Physical activity: The rest of the calories you get from food sources fuel your actual work. This includes both your regular assignments and your exercises. Therefore, the complete number of calories expected to cover this class can shift extraordinarily from one day to another and from one individual to the next. Your body gets calories from the food varieties you eat and

uses them to fuel basal metabolic rate, absorption, and physical activity.

You need a calorie deficit to lose weight

When your body's quick energy needs are met, any overabundance of energy is stored for sometime later. Some of it is stored as glycogen (Carbohydrates) in your muscles and liver, and its remainder will be stored as fat. In this way, on the off chance that you eat a greater number of calories than your body needs, you will put on weight, generally from fat. Then again, if the calories you get from your diet are inadequate to cover your quick requirements, your body is compelled to draw on its energy stores to redress. This state, known as being in a "calorie deficit" makes you get fitter, generally from your muscle-to-fat ratio. Be that as it may, remember when excessive calorie shortage happens from dietary limitations or weighty activity, your body will likewise pull from protein stores, breakdown of muscle as well as consuming muscle to fat ratio for fuel. This concept of maintaining a healthy balance of calories has been proven time and time again, and it holds whether your calories come from carbohydrates, fat, or protein. To lose weight, you always need to burn a greater number of calories than you eat. This can happen through a blend of activity and eating a fair diet and food with some moderation.

The most effective ways to monitor what you eat

If you're keen on counting calories, there are multiple approaches. All include recording what you eat, whether on paper, on the web, or in a portable application. The strategy you pick doesn't exactly make any difference, so it's best to pick the one you like. Using scales and measuring cups can likewise be beneficial for assisting you with measuring food portions all the more precisely.

You could likewise need to have a go at using the following visual rules to gauge your piece sizes. They're less accurate but helpful if you have limited admittance to a scale or measuring cups:

- 1 cup: a baseball or your close hand (suitable for raw or cooked vegetables)
- 3 ounces (90 grams): a deck of cards or the size and thickness of the palm of your hand less the fingers (suitable for estimating meat, poultry, and fish)
- 1 tablespoon (15 mL): a lipstick or the size of your thumb (can quantify nut spreads)
- 1 teaspoon (5 mL): at the tip of your finger (can be used to measure the oils and different fats)

Finally, focusing on counting calories just permits you to assess your diet from a quantitative perspective. It doesn't say much about how good the food is that you eat. With regards to health, 100 calories from apples will influence your health uniquely in contrast to 100 calories from doughnuts. Therefore, it's important to try not to pick food solely based on its calorie content. Instead, ensure you likewise think about their nutrient and mineral substance. You can do this by filling your diet with whole, minimally processed food sources, like fruits, vegetables, whole grains, lean proteins, nuts/seeds, and beans/vegetables. To count your calories most precisely, use a food journal together with scales or measuring cups.

The proper calorie intake for males and females of various ages

Calorie prerequisites

Gender	Age	Calorie intake
Little kids	2-8 years	1,000-1,400
Teenagers	2-8 years	1,000-2,000
Females	9-13 years	1,400-2,200
Male	9-13 years	1,600-2,600
Grown-up women	14-30 years	1,800-2,400
Grown-up men	14-30 years	2,800-3,200
Older women	30 years and over	1,600-2,400
Older men	30 years and over,	2,000-3,000

The health of your day-to-day calories is additionally essential. Food varieties that give primarily calories and very little sustenance are known as "none calories." Examples of food varieties that give no calories include cakes, treats, and doughnuts.

Processed meats, caffeinated beverages, and soft drinks, natural product drinks with added sugar, frozen yogurt, chips and fries.
Pizza, soft drinks. Nonetheless, it's the kind of food as well as the fixings that make it nutritious.

Are there downsides to counting calories?

Even though following your calorie intake can be a viable tool for weight loss, it probably won't be reasonable for everybody. Specifically, it may not be recommended for those with a background of disordered eating, as it could encourage an undesirable relationship with food and deteriorate side effects. According to a research review affecting 105 individuals determined to have a dietary problem, 75% revealed using an internet-based device to count their calories and 73% noticed that they felt this added to their dietary problem. In another study, counting calories and self-weighing all the more of the time was linked to increased eating disorder seriousness among undergraduates. A few studies have had similar discoveries, which suggest that using calorie or fitness trackers or weighing your food, may cause some people to develop unhealthy eating habits. In this manner, if you find that counting your calories or following your food consumption causes sensations of culpability, disgrace, or tension, stopping these practices might be ideal.

Practicing natural eating, which includes paying attention to your body and eating when you feel hungry, may likewise be a superior option for those with a history of disordered eating. Calorie counting may exacerbate eating disorders, cause side effects in some people, and exacerbate an unhealthy relationship with food. The reality is that to lose weight, you need to eat fewer calories than you consume. Certain individuals can do this without really counting calories. Others observe that counting calories is a viable approach to make and keep up with this shortfall intentionally. Those keen on checking calories should keep in mind that not all calories are the same with regards to influence on health, as well as different variables that influence weight loss like hunger and hormones. Subsequently, try to build your menu around minimal process, nutrient-rich food instead of basing your food decisions on calories alone. Moreover, remember that counting calories could add to an unfortunate relationship with food, particularly for those with a history of eating disorders. If you find that tracking your calorie consumption sets off any negative feelings like responsibility or shame, consider other practices instead, like intuitive eating.

What are Nutrients?

Nutrients are substances expected by the body to carry out its essential roles. Since the human body does not synthesize or produce the majority of nutrients, we must consume them. Three fundamental functions are performed by nutrients: They either regulate chemical processes in the body, provide energy, or contribute to the structure of the body. These essential functions enable us to move, eliminate waste, respire (breathe), grow, and reproduce, as well as recognize and respond to our surroundings.

There are six types of nutrients that the body needs to work and stay healthy overall. They are lipids, proteins, starches, water, nutrients, and minerals. The body needs nutrients from nutritious foods. Food sources may likewise contain an assortment of non-supplements. Some non-supplements, for example, as cell reinforcements (tracked down in many plant food varieties) are valuable to the body, though others like normal poisons (normal in some plant food varieties) or added substances (like specific colors and additives tracked down in handled food sources) are possibly unsafe.

The Macronutrients

Macronutrients or "macros," are a group of nutrients that give your body energy and the components it needs to maintain its structure and functions. The nutrients your body requires in large quantities to operate properly are known as macronutrients. Macronutrients include Carbohydrates, protein, and fat. They're required in moderately larger amounts than other nutrients. In spite of the fact that there are recommended ranges for macronutrient intake, your needs differ based on your circumstances.

The three primary macronutrients are fat, protein, and carbohydrates. They're viewed as essential nutrients, meaning your body either can't make them or cannot make enough of them.

For instance, proteins provide essential amino acids, while fats contain essential fatty acids. Your body uses these components for specific functions.

Macronutrients also contain energy as calories. Carbs are the main energy source, but your body can utilize other macronutrients for energy if necessary.

The calorie content of each macronutrient is:

- Carbs: 4 calories for each gram
- Protein: 4 calories for each gram
- Fat: 9 calories for each gram.

The Macronutrients are carbon-based intensifiers that can be metabolically processed into cell energy through changes in their substance bonds. The synthetic energy is changed over into cell energy known as ATP, which is used by the body to perform work and lead essential capabilities.

How much energy an individual consumes each day comes basically from the 3 macronutrients. Food energy is estimated in kilocalories. For convenience, food names express how much energy in food is in "calories," implying that every calorie is duplicated by 1,000 to rise to a kilocalorie. (Note: Using logical phrasing, "Calorie" (with a capital "C") is identical to a kilocalorie. Therefore, 1 kilocalorie = 1 Calorie - 1000 calories

Water is likewise a macronutrient as the body needs it in large sums, yet dissimilar to the next macronutrient, it doesn't contain carbon or yield energy.

It is important to note that drinking alcohol likewise contributes energy (calories) to the diet of 7 kilocalories/gram, so it should be included in daily energy usage. In any case, alcohol isn't viewed as a "Nutrient" since it doesn't add to essential body capabilities and contains substances that must be broken down and discharged from the body to forestall poisonous effects.

A. Carbohydrates: Carbohydrates are atoms made out of carbon, hydrogen, and oxygen that give energy to the body. The significant food wellsprings of carbs are milk, grains, natural products, and bland vegetables, similar to potatoes. Non-dull vegetables likewise contain sugars yet in lesser amounts. Carbohydrates are comprehensively characterized into two structures in light of their substance structure: basic carbs (frequently called straightforward sugars) and complex carbs.

Straightforward carbs comprise a couple of fundamental sugar units connected. Their logical names are "monosaccharides" (1 sugar unit) and disaccharides (2 sugar units). They are separated and consumed rapidly in the gastrointestinal system and give a quick eruption of energy to the body. Instances of basic sugars incorporate the disaccharide sucrose, the sort of sugar you would have in a bowl on the morning meal table, and the monosaccharide glucose, the most widely recognized kind of fuel for most living beings including people. Glucose is the essential sugar that blood courses to give energy to cells. The expressions "glucose" and "blood glucose" can be filled in for one another.

Complex carbs are long chains of sugar units that can connect in a straight seat or an extended chain. During assimilation, the body separates edible complex starches into straightforward sugars, for the most part, glucose. Glucose is then retained in the circulation system and shipped to every one of our cells where it is put away, used to make energy, or used to fabricate macromolecules. Fiber is likewise a mind-boggling starch, however, it can't be separated by stomach-related catalysts in the human digestive tract. Accordingly, it goes through the gastrointestinal system undigested except if the microorganisms that possess the colon or internal organ separate it.

One gram of absorbable carbs yields 4 kilocalories of energy for the cells in the body to perform work. As well as giving energy and filling in as building blocks for greater macromolecules, sugars are fundamental for the legitimate working of the sensory system, heart, and kidneys. As referenced, glucose can be put away in the body for some time later. In people, the capacity atom of sugars is called glycogen, and in plants, it is known as starch. Glycogen and starch are complicated sugars.

B. Lipids: Lipids are likewise a group of particles made out of carbon, hydrogen, and oxygen, however dissimilar to sugars, they are insoluble in water. Lipids are tracked down prevalently in margarine, oils, meats, dairy items, nuts, and seeds, and in many processed foods. The three principal sorts of lipids are fatty oils (triacylglycerols), phospholipids, and sterols. The principal occupation of triacylglycerols is to give or store energy. Lipids give more energy per gram than sugars (9 kilocalories for every gram of lipids versus 4 kilocalories for each gram of starches).

Notwithstanding energy stockpiling, lipids act as a significant part of cell layers, encompass and safeguard organs (in fat-putting away tissues), and give protection to support temperature guidelines. Phospholipids and sterols have to some degree different compound construction and are utilized to manage numerous different capabilities in the body.

C. Proteins: Proteins are macromolecules made out of chains of essential subunits called amino acids. Carbon, oxygen, hydrogen, and nitrogen make up amino acids. Food wellsprings of proteins incorporate meats, dairy items, fish, and a wide range of plant-based food varieties, most remarkably soy. The word protein comes from a Greek word signifying "of essential significance," which is a well-suited portrayal of these macronutrients; they are likewise referred to conversationally as the "workhorses" of life. Proteins give the fundamental construction to bones, muscles, skin, catalysts, and chemicals and assume a part in leading the majority of the substance responses that happen in the body. Researchers gauge that more than 100,000 unique proteins exist inside the human body. The hereditary codes in DNA are essentially protein recipes that decide the request wherein 20 unique amino acids are bound together to make a large number of explicit proteins. Since amino acids contain carbon, they can be involved by the body for energy and supply 4 kilocalories of energy for each gram; but giving energy isn't protein's most significant capability.

D. Water: There is another supplement that we should have in huge amounts: water. Water doesn't contain carbon, however, it is made out of two hydrogen iotas and one oxygen particle for each atom of water. More than 60% of your all-out body weight is water. Without water, nothing could be shipped in or out of the body, substance responses wouldn't happen, organs wouldn't be padded, and internal heat levels would broadly vary. By and large, a grown-up polishes off a little more than two liters of water each day from both eating food varieties and drinking fluids. Since water is so basic for life's essential cycles, absolute water admission and results are especially significant.

The Micronutrients

The term micronutrients refers to minerals and vitamins, which can be divided into macrominerals, minor elements, and water- and fat-soluble vitamins. A satisfactory amount of micronutrients often implies aiming for a balanced diet. Macronutrients, on the other hand, incorporate proteins, fats and carbohydrates. Micronutrients are one of the major groups of nutrients your body requires. They include vitamins and minerals.

Vitamins are important for energy production, blood clotting, immune function, and other functions. Meanwhile, minerals play a significant role in growth, bone health, fluid balance, and a few other processes. Your body needs fewer micronutrients than macronutrients, which are more abundant. That is the reason they're labelled "micro."

Humans must obtain micronutrients from food since your body can't produce vitamins and minerals generally. That is the reason they're referred to as essential nutrients.

Vitamins are organic compounds made by plants and animals that can be broken down by heat, air, or acid. Then again, minerals are inorganic, exist in soil or water, and cannot be broken down.

At the point when you eat, you consume the vitamin that plants and animals created or the minerals they absorbed. The micronutrient content of every food is unique, so it's ideal to eat different food varieties to get an adequate number of vitamins and minerals. An adequate intake of all micronutrients is important for optimal health, as each vitamin and mineral plays a specific role in your body. Vitamins and minerals are crucial for body development, immune function, mental health, and numerous other important functions. Depending on their function, certain micronutrients also play a role in preventing and tackling diseases.

Aside from macronutrients, the micronutrients are not a source of energy (calories) for the body. Rather they play a part as cofactors or parts of catalysts (i.e., coenzymes) that work with synthetic responses in the body. They are associated with all parts of the body's capabilities from delivering energy, to processing supplements, to building macromolecules.

1. **Minerals:** Minerals are strong inorganic substances that structure gems and are arranged relying upon the amount of them we want. Minor elements, like molybdenum, selenium, zinc, iron, and iodine, are just expected in a couple of milligrams or less. Macrominerals, like calcium, magnesium, potassium, sodium, and phosphorus, are expected in many milligrams. Numerous minerals are basic for compound capability, while others are used to keep up with liquid equilibrium, fabricate bone tissue, orchestrate chemicals, send nerve motivations, contract and loosen up muscles, and safeguard against hurtful free extremists in the body that can cause medical conditions like malignant growth.

2. **Vitamin:** The thirteen vitamins are classified as either water-solvent or fat-dissolvable. The water-dissolvable nutrients are L-ascorbic acid and all the B nutrients, which include thiamine, riboflavin, niacin, pantothenic corrosive, pyridoxine, biotin, folate, and cobalamin. A, D, E, and K are some of the fat-soluble vitamins. Vitamins are expected to carry out numerous roles in the body, for example, aiding energy creation, making red platelets, orchestrating bone tissue, and supporting ordinary vision, sensory system capability, and safe framework capability.

Lack of nutrients can cause serious medical conditions and even passing. For instance, a lack of niacin causes an illness called pellagra, which was normal in the mid-20th hundred years in certain parts of America. The normal signs and side effects of pellagra are known as the "4D's — looseness of the bowels, dermatitis, dementia, and demise." Until researchers found that better eating regimens let the signs and side effects free from pellagra, many individuals with the sickness wound up hospitalized in psychiatric hospitals anticipating passing. Different nutrients were likewise found to forestall specific issues and illnesses like scurvy (L-ascorbic acid), night visual impairment (vitamin A), and rickets (vitamin D).

Water-dissolvable

Thiamin (B1).	Coenzyme, and energy digestion help.
Riboflavin (B2).	Coenzyme, and energy digestion help.
Niacin (B3).	Coenzyme, and energy digestion help.
Pantothenic corrosive (B5).	Coenzyme, and energy digestion help.
Pyridoxine (B6)	Coenzyme, an amino corrosive combination, helps.
Biotin (B7)	Coenzyme, amino corrosive and unsaturated fat digestion.
Folate (B9)	Coenzyme,

	fundamental for development.
Cobalamin (B12)	Coenzyme, red platelet combination.

How to balance micro vs. macro nutrients

If you're eating a balanced diet like the Paleo diet that incorporates different plant and animal foods, carbs, saturated fats, and protein and you feel much better, then, at that point, you probably don't have to stress over your macronutrient and micronutrient consumption. However, one supplement to be aware of on a Paleo diet is calcium, since Paleo confines dairy items. However, there are alternate ways of getting more calcium in your diet if you can't endure dairy, including green leaf vegetables, cross veggies, and canned bone-in fish.

For macronutrients, many dieticians and nutritionists advise eating a meal that should be composed of half of the good vegetables and a small number of fruits. If you prefer 25% of the protein, a quarter of the bland vegetables, whole grains, or whole fruit.

Add a limited quantity of saturated fats, frequently as healthy cooking oil. Eating a meal three times each day that generally follows this example should get you to the required rates of sugars, fats, and protein that were recommended earlier. Mixing the range of those food sources (consider eating every one of the shades of the rainbow) should supply each of the micronutrients you want too.

Understanding balanced diet

A balanced diet gives your body the nutrients it requires to accurately work. To get the nourishment you want, the vast majority of your everyday calories ought to come from new fruits, new vegetables, whole grains, vegetables, nuts, and lean proteins. A good meal furnishes the body with every one of the nutrients it requires to keep up with typical development and fix capabilities.

A custom-made pizza with a wholemeal base and a lot of new veggies on top might be a solid decision. Interestingly, pre-made pizzas and other exceptionally processed foods often contain void calories.

To keep up with great health, limit your intake of void calories and on second thought try to get your calories from food sources that are rich in other nutrients.

Find a way to resist the desire for less nutritious food varieties.

Calories are a proportion of energy that foods supply. The quantity of calories you want will depend upon your sex, age, and movement level.

Reasons why a balanced diet is significant

A balanced diet supplies the nutrients your body needs to successfully work. Without adjusted sustenance, your body is more inclined to illness, contamination, exhaustion, and low execution.

Children who don't get an adequate number of good foods might confront growth and formative issues, unfortunate work execution, and regular contaminations.

They can also foster unfortunate dietary patterns that might continue into adulthood.

Without working out, they'll likewise have a higher risk of obesity and different illnesses that make up metabolic conditions, for example, type 2 diabetes and high blood pressure.

Based on research, 4 of the main 10 driving reasons for death in the US are highly linked to eating less. Among them are type 2 diabetes, heart disease, and stroke. Concentrate on good meal plans for children.

Your body needs nutrients to remain healthy, and food supplies essential nutrients that prevent us from becoming ill.

Types of food to eat for a perfect balanced diet

A solid, balanced diet will generally include the following supplements:

- Vitamins, minerals, and antioxidants.
- Sugars, including Carbohydrates and fiber, protein, and solid fats.

A balanced diet will include different food varieties from the following groups:

- Fruits
- vegetables
- grains
- Journal
- protein foods

Examples of protein-rich food items include meat, eggs, fish, beans, nuts, and vegetables.

People who follow a vegetarian diet will focus on plant-based food varieties. They will not eat meat, fish, or dairy, yet their eating routine will include different things that give equal nutrients.

Tofu and beans, for instance, are plant-based sources of protein. Certain individuals are narrow-minded of dairy however can in any case create a reasonable diet by picking various nutrient-rich alternatives.

Fruit products

Fruits are nutritious, they make a scrumptious tidbit or pastry, and they can produce a sweet tooth. Neighbourhood fruits that are in season are fresher and give a larger amount of nutrients than imported fruits.

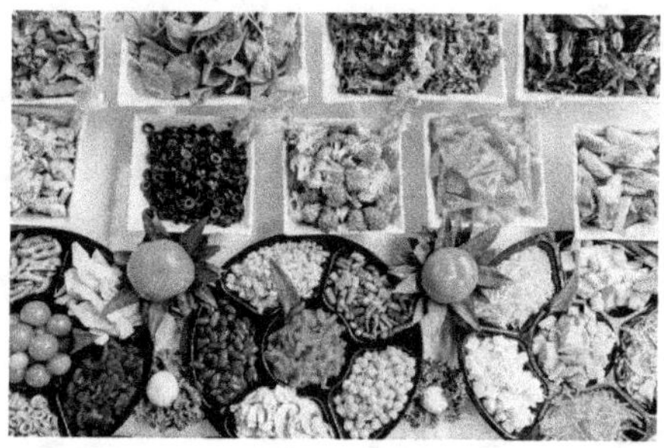

Fruits are high in sugar, however, this sugar is normal. It's not like candy and various sweet treats, fruit additionally gives fiber and different nutrients. This implies they're less inclined to cause a sugar spike and they'll help the body's stock of essential vitamins, minerals, and antioxidants.

If you have diabetes, your PCP or dietitian can help you with which fruit to choose, the amount to eat, and when.

Vegetables

Vegetables are a critical source of essential vitamins, minerals, and antioxidants. Eat various vegetables with various varieties for a full scope of supplements.

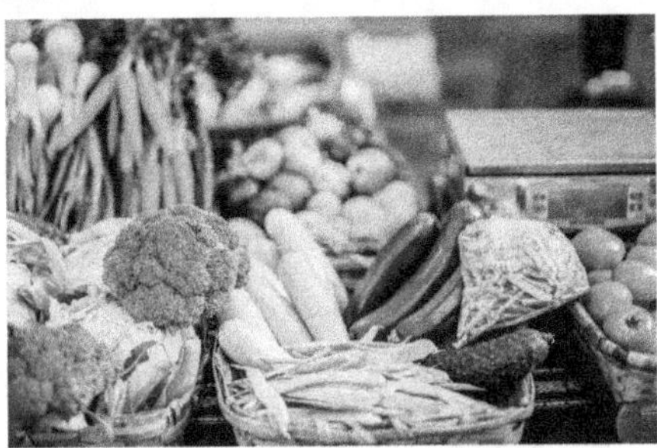

Feeble, Leafy greens are an amazing source of numerous nutrients. They include:

- spinach
- kale
- green beans
- broccoli
- collard greens
- Swiss chard

Also, random vegetables are most times lower in cost and easy to prepare. Use them in the following ways:

- As a side dish
- Cooked on a plate with a splash of olive oil
- Serving as the foundation for soups, stews, and pasta dishes

- As a serving of mixed greens
- In juices and smoothies.

Proteins

Meats and beans are an essential source of protein, which is fundamental for wound recuperation and muscle support and improvement, among different capabilities.

1. **Animal-base protein**

Healthy animal-based protein choices include red meats, like hamburgers and lamb.

poultry, like chicken and turkey.

fish, including salmon, sardines, and other sleek fish.

Processed meats and red meats might increase the risk of malignant growth and different infections,

1. **Plant-based protein**

Nuts, beans, and soy items are great sources of protein, fiber, and different nutrients.

Examples include lentils, beans, peas, almonds, sunflower seeds, and pecans.

Tofu, tempeh, and other soy-based items are amazing sources of protein and are great options rather than meat. Go for tofu and tempeh.

Food Journal

Journal items give fundamental nutrients, including: protein, calcium, and vitamin D.

They additionally contain fat. If you're trying to limit your fat intake, reduced fat choices may be ideal. Your primary care physician can assist you with choosing.

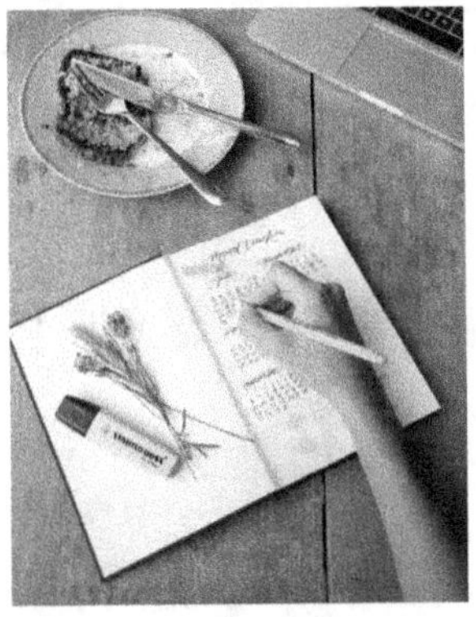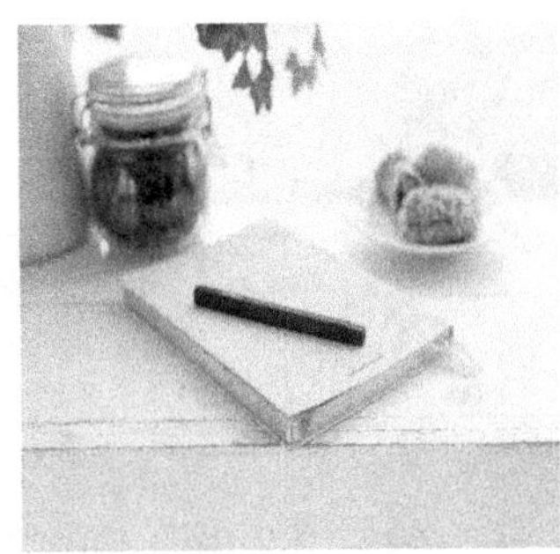

For those following a vegetarian diet, numerous sans-dairy milks and other dairy options are presently accessible, produced using: flax seed, almonds and cashews, soy, oats, and coconut.

These are frequently strengthened with calcium and different supplements, making them phenomenal options in contrast to dairy from cows. Some have added sugar, so always read the label while picking. Look for almond and soy milk.

Fats and oils

Fat is fundamental for energy and cell wellbeing, however, an excess of fat can increase calories above what the body needs and may prompt weight gain.

Previously, rules have suggested keeping away from saturated fats, because of worries that they would raise cholesterol levels.

Researchers propose that to some degree supplanting with unsaturated fats brings down cardiovascular disease and that some saturated fat should be in the diet around 10% or less of calories.

Trans fats, nonetheless, should in any case be avoided. Consumable fat includes vegetable oils and fish oils.

Fats to avoid are spread, cheddar, and weighty cream.

Fats to lose include trans fats that are used in many processed and pre-made foods, like doughnuts.

Most specialists believe olive oil to be a healthy fat, particularly additional virgin olive oil, which is the most unprocessed type. Pan-fried food varieties are many times high in calories yet low in dietary benefits, so you should eat them occasionally.

A good diet contains food sources from the following groups: fruits, vegetables, grains, and protein.

A balanced diet comprises the nutrients and food groups listed above, however, you want to adjust them, as well. A convenient method for recollecting the amount of every nutritional group to eat is the plate strategy which is:

- using leafy foods to fill a portion of your plate.
- filling a little more than one-quarter with grains.
- filling just a little of one quarter with protein food sources.
- including dairy on the side (or a nondairy substitution).

However, individual necessities will change, so the USDA likewise gives an intelligent apparatus, "MyPlate Plan" where you can enter your subtleties to figure out your requirements.

Hold back nothing for your food to come from products of the soil, around one-quarter to be protein, and one-quarter whole grains and carbohydrates.

A significant and balanced diet is typically one that thatcontains a lot of new, plant-based food varieties and limits the intake of processed food varieties.

If you have inquiries regarding your diet or feel that you want to lose weight or change your dietary patterns, the following processes previously above will be effective.

Food varieties to avoid

Foods to stay away from or limit on a healthy balanced diet include:

- Highly processed foods
- Refined grains (oats) like maida, white bread, sewing, noodles, and pasta.
- Added sugar and salt
- Red and processed meat
- Alcohol
- Trans fat, spread cheese, and cakes.

What's good for one individual may not be appropriate for another.

For Instance, whole wheat flour can be a healthy substance for some individuals yet it is good for those with a gluten bigotry,

Essential Vitamins and Their Food Sources

Vitamins are essential nutrients that play a crucial role in maintaining overall health and well-being. They are organic compounds required in small quantities for various physiological functions in the body. While a balanced diet typically provides an adequate amount of vitamins, it is essential to understand their sources to ensure proper intake. Here is a comprehensive overview of essential vitamins and their food sources.

Vitamins	**Food source**
Vitamin A	Carrots, sweet potatoes, spinach, kale, apricots, mangoes, eggs, liver, and dairy products.
Vitamin B1 (Thiamine)	Whole grains, fortified cereals, legumes, nuts, seeds, pork, and organ meats.
Vitamin B2 (Riboflavin)	Dairy products, lean meats, eggs, green leafy vegetables, almonds, and mushrooms.
Vitamin B3 (Niacin)	Meat, poultry, fish, whole grains, legumes, nuts, and seeds.
Vitamin B5 (Pantothenic Acid)	Meat, poultry, fish, whole grains,

	avocados, broccoli, and mushrooms.
Vitamin B6	Poultry, fish, organ meats, bananas, potatoes, chickpeas, and fortified cereals.
Vitamin B7 (Biotin)	Eggs, organ meats, nuts, seeds, sweet potatoes, and dairy products.
Vitamin B9 (Folate)	Leafy green vegetables, legumes, asparagus, citrus fruits, avocados, and fortified grains.
Vitamin B12	Meat, poultry, fish, dairy products, eggs, and fortified plant-based milk.
Vitamin C	Citrus fruits (oranges, lemons, grapefruits),

	strawberries, kiwi, bell peppers, broccoli, and tomatoes.
Vitamin D	Fatty fish (salmon, mackerel, sardines), fortified dairy products, egg yolks, and sunlight exposure.
Vitamin E	Nuts, seeds, vegetable oils (such as sunflower and olive oil), avocados, and spinach.
Vitamin K	Leafy green vegetables (kale, spinach, broccoli), Brussels sprouts, cabbage, and liver.
Vitamin H (Biotin)	Eggs, organ meats, nuts, seeds, sweet potatoes, and dairy products.

Vitamin P (Bioflavonoids)	Citrus fruits, berries, grapes, cherries, onions, and green tea.

A varied and balanced diet consisting of fruits, vegetables, whole grains, lean proteins, and healthy fats is the best way to obtain the necessary vitamins and minerals. Whole foods are generally the preferred way to obtain vitamins, in certain cases, supplements may be recommended by healthcare professionals to address specific deficiencies.

Chapter 2
Healthy diet

A solid healthy diet is a diet that maintains or improves general well-being. A sound healthy diet furnishes the body with nutrients, liquid, macronutrients, such as protein, micronutrients like vitamins, and sufficient fiber and food energy. A healthy diet during all phases of life is crucial to prevent some non-communicable chronic diseases (NCDs), like obesity and diabetes. Along with physical activity, a healthy diet is fundamental to achieving "sustainable health", which is defined as "healthy and dynamic ageing avoiding the risk of diseases. Prevention of cardiovascular disease and its risk factors, such as diabetes and obesity, begins with a healthy diet. Eating various fresh and whole foods consistently can help you get the right amount of essential nutrients to lower your risk of CVD and help you live a more active life. A healthy diet is particularly important for small kids, as it supports their development and sets standards for them to follow later in life. However healthy eating is not always up to the individual all of the time. According to research, almost one in four individuals around the world lack access to safe, nutritious, and adequate food. People are greatly influenced by their social surroundings and economic circumstances, and for some, a healthy diet is just difficult to access. The wide availability of processed and ultra-processed food varieties, urbanization, and changing ways of life have additionally contributed to unhealthy changes in dietary patterns, especially in low and middle-income countries.

Individual responsibility can only have its full impact when people have access to a healthy lifestyle and are supported to go with healthy choices. Supportive environments and networks are essential in shaping people's dietary habits and inclinations. To eat healthier, begin by making small changes. Make every meal or snack contain nutrient-dense food, and be sure to stay away from processed food.

How to start a healthy diet

Many people want to start eating more nutritively and in a healthier way. At the point when your diet contains a lot of excessively processed food, high-fat food, or foods high in sugar, you increase your risk for a variety of chronic health issues. Then again, a nutritious, well-balanced diet can support your immune system, and sound development, and lessen your risk for obesity, diabetes, and high blood pressure. Make small changes to your diet throughout a few weeks rather than numerous drastic changes at once, and you'll be able to sustain a better healthier way of eating and enjoy the health benefits of a healthy diet.

Plan and Prep

Set a goal for yourself

Beginning a healthier diet is a great general goal; however, to make your goal more sensible and possible, you'll need to be more specific about what you want out of a "healthy diet.

1. It may be helpful to first think about your current diet. What's unhealthy about it? Do you have to eat more green vegetables? Do you need to hydrate? Would it be a good idea for you to snack less?

2. Write up the list of the things you need to change, add, or stop about your ongoing dieting. Use these ideas to form numerous small goals to help you reach a healthier diet.

3. The most effective way to reach any goal is, to begin with one or two very small changes. Trying to update your entire diet in a couple of days probably won't work well. Choose something small to work on every week. In the long run, you'll have much greater success. Start a food journal. After you've come up with a few goals and how you can accomplish them, think about starting a food

journal. This will serve as a method to follow and assess your progress.

4. Compose every one of your objectives in your food diary. You can survey them depending on the situation or change them as you keep on making changes to your eating routine.

5. Also, track all your food in general and drinks in your food journal. This will help physically see what's absent from your diet or what you're eating too much of. Make sure to write out each breakfast, lunch, dinner, nibbles (even a couple of snacks), and drinks you consume over the day. This will be a better resource if you are more precise. Each week in your food journal, record the change you want to work on. For instance, "This week, I will drink 7 glasses of water every day." Toward the week's end, revisit your diary to check whether you've completed this goal.

6. There are numerous applications accessible to download on your smartphone that can help you track calories, exercise, and even how much water you drink.

Make a meal plan.

A meal plan is an incredible tool when you're trying to follow any new diet plan. These plans are your aid and blueprint for your seven-day stretch of meals and snacks.

1. Meal plans can help you stay organized and on track consistently. You'll know precisely the exact thing you will have and on what day. This way you can go to the supermarket with a specific list, only purchasing what you plan to use in your meal for the week. You can likewise plan ahead of time for busy days for instance, if you realize you'll be extremely occupied and work late on Thursday, make something on Wednesday that you can easily reheat and have leftover on Thursday.

2. Also, write up the corresponding basic food item list to your meal plans. This will help you get in and out of the supermarket and ensure you have all of the necessary ingredients at home to make all of your meals.

3. Try not to skip meals. On the off chance that you skip meals, make sure to schedule a meal or a healthy snack for yourself at least every four hours. Skipping meals is more

likely to lead to voraciously consuming food later, which contributes to weight gain.

Meal prep in your leisure time.

In a situation where you're busy and have little time to make a meal from scratch, meal prep will be the key to following your new healthy diet.

1. Meal prep helps you get a lot of the work of cooking without any preparation or cooking at home out of the way during your free time. At the point when it's time for dinner on a busy weeknight, you should have most or even all of the cooking already done.

2. Plan to prepare your meals on one or more days during the week when you have some free time. Review your meal plan and basic food item list and attempt to track down ways to get some cooking done.

3. Meal prep is flexible. You can prepare a full dinner ahead of time so you simply need to reheat the night you need to eat it, or you can do washing or chopping of meat or marinating vegetables so you can quickly prepare food the night before. Also, consider buying foods that require less prep work in any case. For instance, you can purchase pre-washed and cut bagged lettuce rather than a whole head of lettuce, frozen vegetables that are heated and served, or

pre-grilled lean protein like grilled chicken
strips.

4. Meal preparation can be an opportunity to
   catch up with people. Ask your partner or
   kids to help you prep while you discuss what
   has been going on in your lives.

What to Eat

Go for a well-balanced diet.

Even though there are different eating styles and
diet plans to follow, the most nutritious is a
well-balanced diet

1. A balanced diet will be different for
   everybody. You'll need to eat the right
   portion for your age, gender, and activity
   level.

2. Additionally, a well-balanced diet highlights
   foods from each nutrition class each day.
   Although many diets recommend giving up
   gluten, or giving up carbs, or even, keeping
   away from dairy, all food groups offer
   beneficial nutrition to everyone. Only stay
   away from certain food groups if you have
   an allergy to them.

3. Also, ensure you have a wide variety of
   foods in your diet. For example, don't
   always in every case choose to eat an apple
   as your afternoon snack. Shift between

apples, bananas, or berries to increase the variety of your diet.

Select lean protein over sources of protein with more fat.

Protein is an essential supplement to any nutritious diet; in any case, choosing leaner protein sources is fitting.

1. Protein is essential for various functions in your body which include providing your body with energy, supporting your lean muscle mass, giving the basis to numerous enzymes and hormones, and providing structure and support for cells.
2. In comparison to proteins with higher fat content, lean protein sources have fewer calories and fat. Some high-fat proteins (mostly from animal sources) are higher in Saturated fat. Focusing on leaner fatty protein decreases your general intake of these types of fat.
3. To get your recommended of protein every day, include a couple of servings at each meal. One serving is around 3 - 4 oz or about the size of the palm of your hand.
4. Lean protein sources include poultry, eggs, low-fat dairy, pork, fish, beans and nuts, and lower-fat beef.

Get a way of including five to nine servings of fruits and vegetables each day.

Fruit and vegetables are an integral part of an energizing healthful diet. These are the foods with a high concentration of vital nutrients. Fruit and vegetables are both genuinely low in calories, yet high in nutrients (making them nutrient-dense foods). They are probably the best sources of fiber, vitamins, minerals, and antioxidants.

1. Consuming five to nine servings of fruits and vegetables every day is typically recommended. So measure out 1 cup of vegetables, 2 cups of leafy greens, and 1/2 cup of fruits to help you meet this recommendation.

2. If you don't regularly eat a lot of fruits or vegetables currently, increasing your intake to five to nine servings daily can be difficult. Find simple methods for getting a few of these essential foods. Try mixing sautéed vegetables into eggs for breakfast, sprinkle yogurt or cottage cheese with fruit, add additional lettuce, tomatoes, and onions to your sandwiches, or have a go at making your mac and cheese recipe with some steamed vegetables.

Pick whole grains over refined grains.

A simple method for increasing your nutrition and eating a healthier diet is by choosing 100% whole grains. These foods are vastly better for you than refined grains.

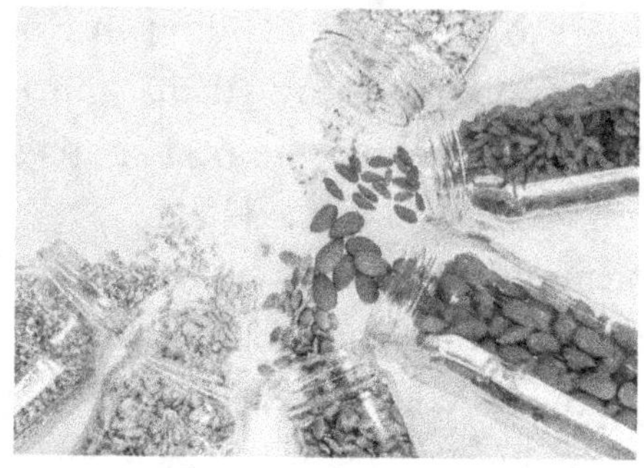

1. 100,% whole grains have each of the three parts of the grain: the germ, bran, and endosperm. They are less processed and contain a lot more nutrients like fiber, protein, and minerals.
2. Refined grains are much more processed than whole grains. They are normally stripped of the bran and microorganism so they are lower in fiber and protein. Avoid foods made with white flour like white pasta, white rice, cakes, chips, and crackers.
3. Include a couple of servings of whole grains every day. Measure out a 1 oz or 1/2 cup serving to help you adhere to proper portion sizes.

4. Try whole grains like quinoa, brown rice, whole wheat pasta, millet, farro, or whole wheat bread and wraps.

Follow the 80/20 rule. Even though you need to follow a healthier diet, enjoying your favorite foods is still appropriate.

Following the 80/20 rule can help you with adhering to a healthy diet while eating more liberal foods with some moderate.

1. Even though eating a nutritious, well-balanced diet is important, eating perfectly healthy consistently until the end of your life is not realistic. People derive a great deal of pleasure from eating and once in a while eating more indulgent foods.
2. Treat yourself to an indulgent dish, glass of alcohol, or larger portion once in a while. This is as yet considered to be normal and healthy dieting; however, just enjoy 20% of the time. More often than not, or 80% of the time, you should be choosing quality foods.

Choose healthy fat sources.

Although fat should be checked in your diet, there are a few types of fat that are especially healthy and provide a variety of health benefits.

1. If you're trying to eat more sources of sound fats, make sure to swap them out for

unhealthy fats. Try not to add more fats,
healthy or not, on top of a diet containing
unhealthy fats.

2. Omega 3 fats and monounsaturated fats are
   both perfect for your body. They have been
   shown to improve cardiovascular health and
   further develop cholesterol levels.

3. The best sources of these healthy fats are
   avocados, olive oil, olives, nuts, nut
   margarine, canola oil, chia seeds, flaxseeds,
   and fatty fish (like salmon, tuna, and
   mackerel). Keep in mind that these may
   likewise have a high-calorie count, so be
   moderate.

4. Many health experts recommend eating fatty
   fish at least two times every week and
   including a daily source of other healthy
   fats.

Drink satisfactory water.

Even though water isn't its nutrition type or nutrient, it is a fundamental part of a healthy diet and a healthy body.

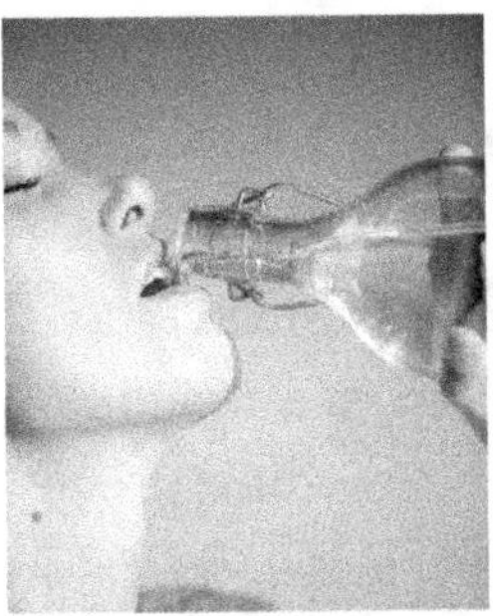

1. Drinking sufficient water consistently helps your body remain hydrated. It's very important to help regulate body temperature, constipation, and blood pressure.
2. It's typically recommended to drink something like eight 8-oz glasses (2 liters) of water each day. However, presently numerous health professionals suggest consuming up to 13 glasses (3 liters) daily.
3. Also on the water, you can try flavored water, decaf unsweetened coffee, and tea. These beverages are no calorie and caffeine-free which are awesome and most hydrating liquids.

What to Avoid

Reduce your intake of sources of added and highly processed sugar.
There are some groups of foods that you should limit and just eat with some restraint. Added sugars are something that should be eaten with some moderation as they often have no dietary benefit.

1. Added sugars are added to specific food varieties during their processing. They offer no nutrition, just extra calories. Furthermore, many studies have shown that a diet high in added sugars can prompt obesity.
2. Many different foods contain added sugars. Try to limit things like breakfast pastries, Cooked, cakes, frozen yogurt, candy, and grains.
3. Also, limit sweetened beverages. In addition to the fact that they are high in added sugars and calories, many people also don't remember to count these kinds of beverages as a source since they don't fill you up as much as food does in terms of calories. You might wind up drinking more calories through these refreshments.
4. The American Heart Affiliation suggests that women consume no more than 6 teaspoons and men consume something like 9 teaspoons of added sugar daily.

Limit sources of unhealthy fats.

In addition to added sugars, you should limit certain gatherings of foods that contain high amounts of fat. Specifically, you need to avoid higher levels of Saturated and trans fat.

1. There has been some discussion about whether or not saturated fat is as dangerous or unhealthy as previously thought. Nonetheless, saturated fat is as yet a fat which means it's very calorie-dense and if eaten in large amounts can in any case lead to weight gain and unfavourable health impacts.

2. You don't have to stay away from every single saturated fat but do eat them with some moderation. Especially foods like full-fat dairy, fatty cuts of beef or pork, stored meats, and other processed meats.

3. Trans fats have been straightforwardly linked to several adverse health effects like raising bad cholesterol levels and bringing down the good kind, increasing your risk for heart disease and stroke, and increasing your risk for developing diabetes. As much as you can, try to avoid these foods. Trans fats are found in various food sources including pastries, cookies, cakes, margarines, pies,

fast food, seared food varieties, fried food, and soy sauce.
4. There is no protected limit for trans fats. When at all possibilities, stay away from these.

Drink a limited amount of alcohol.
If you decide to drink, do such with some moderation. Moderate amounts of alcohol generally don't pose a health risk for many people.
1. If you drink a larger amount of alcohol (multiple servings daily), you might increase your risk of hypertension, liver disease, heart disease, stroke, and depression.
2. Unlike some certain foods, there is a particular definition of moderate alcohol consumption. Women shouldn't drink more than one serving daily and men ought to consume not more than two each day.
3. If you do drink, consider skipping mixed beverages that are blended in with sweetened beverages. Order fruit juices as these contain extra calories and added sugars.
4. One serving is equivalent to a 12-oz brew, 5 oz of wine, or 1.5 oz of alcohol.

Chapter 3
Debunking Dieting Myths

Dieting has become a widespread practice in the pursuit of health and weight management. Unfortunately, amidst the information, numerous myths and misconceptions about dieting have emerged. These myths often lead to confusion and unrealistic expectations, hindering individuals from achieving their health goals effectively. In this short piece, we'll debunk some of the most prevalent dieting myths to promote a more balanced and evidence-based approach to nutrition and weight loss.

A diet myth is a guidance that becomes famous without realities to back it up. About weight reduction, numerous mainstream views are legends and others are just incompletely evident. Here are a few realities to assist you with figuring out what you hear.

MYTH: People are born with a fast metabolism and some are born with slow metabolism

Metabolism is the collective term for the chemical processes that turn food into energy in the body's cells. Our bodies require this energy to move, think, and develop. Each cycle in your body requires energy. Processing food, breathing, and syphoning oxygen to your blood all include synthetic cycles that keep you alive and working.

The base measure of energy you want to proceed with this large number of cycles is known as basal metabolic rate (BMR). Frequently, when individuals allude to an "inability to burn calories," they're alluding to a low BMR.

Certain individuals guarantee to have been brought into the world with "quick digestion." There is a hereditary part to digestion, yet your way of life and well-being propensities bigger affect your digestion than you might suspect. The main variable that influences your digestion rate is bulk. The more muscle you have, the more productively your digestion works. For instance, men might have quicker digestion systems because men will generally have more bulk and less muscle versus fat than ladies. Furthermore, people will quite often lose weight as they age, which makes sense as to why individuals experience an eased back digestion as they age.

Certain individuals are guaranteed to experience difficulty losing weight given an "inability to burn calories." Your dietary patterns do influence your digestion, however truly surprisingly nuanced.

At the point when you go on a crash, abstain from food, or seriously confine your calorie consumption, your body needs to track down energy someplace. Subsequently, your body might begin separating muscles for energy. At the point when you lose bulk, your digestion eases back. After you stop an accident diet, you might bounce back and restore weight rapidly, because you've lost bulk.

The most effective way to shed pounds is to consume a greater number of calories than you consume while meeting the caloric requirements of your BMR. This could mean you get in shape all the more leisurely however, it will be simpler to keep the load off on the off chance that you don't consume bulk. Assuming you experience difficulty shedding pounds, you might be mistakenly assessing the number of calories that you're consuming. Except if you measure your part estimates, it tends to be not difficult to overconsume solid yet calorically thick food sources, like nuts, peanut butter, or olive oils.

In uncommon cases, a hidden condition might influence your digestion, like hypothyroidism (underactive thyroid organ) or Cushing's disorder. Working with your medical care supplier to oversee basic circumstances can help you accomplish and keep a solid weight.

The possibility that individuals are brought into the world with intrinsically quick or sub-optimal abilities to burn calories is a distortion. While hereditary qualities assume a part in metabolic rate, various variables, for example, age, bulk, diet, actual work, and hormonal equilibrium, all in all, impact a singular's digestion. Digestion can likewise be adjusted and impacted over the long haul through way-of-life changes. Consequently, it's incorrect to credit digestion exclusively to hereditary qualities, as a complicated interaction of different variables decides a person's metabolic rate.

MYTH: All calories are equal

The calorie is an estimation of energy. All calories have a similar energy content. Nonetheless, this doesn't imply that all calorie sources affect your weight.

Various food varieties go through various metabolic pathways and can affect hunger and the chemicals that manage your body weight. For instance, a protein calorie isn't equivalent to a fat or carb calorie.

Supplanting carbs and fat with protein can help your digestion and lessen hunger and desires, all while improving the capability of some weight-managing chemicals. Additionally, calories from entire food sources like organic products will quite often be substantially more filling than calories from refined food sources, like sweets. Not all calorie sources meaningfully affect your well-being and weight. For instance, protein can increment digestion, diminish hunger, and work on the capability of weight-directing chemicals.

MYTH: Weight loss is a linear process

Getting in shape is generally not a direct cycle, as certain individuals naturally suspect. Occasionally and weeks you might get in shape, while during others you might acquire a smidgen. This isn't a reason to worry. It's typical for body weight to vacillate all over by a couple of pounds. For instance, you might be conveying more food in your stomach-related framework or clutching more water than expected. This is considerably more articulated in ladies, as water weight can vacillate essentially during the period. However long the general pattern is going downwards, regardless of the amount it varies, you will in any case prevail with regards to getting more fit over the long haul. Getting in shape can consume a large chunk of the day. The cycle is for the most part not straight, as your weight will in general vacillate all over by limited quantities.

MYTH: Supplements can assist you to lose weight

The weight reduction supplement industry is monstrous. Different organizations guarantee that their enhancements make sensational impacts, yet they're seldom exceptionally viable when examined. The principal reason that enhancements work for certain individuals is a self-influenced consequence. Individuals succumb to the promoting strategies and believe that the enhancements should assist them with shedding pounds, so they become more aware of what they eat. All things considered, a couple of enhancements humbly affect weight reduction. The best ones might assist you with shedding a limited quantity of weight for more than a while. Most enhancements for weight reduction are incapable. All that can assist you with losing a touch of weight, probably.

MYTH: Obesity is about willpower, not biology

It is wrong to say that your weight is about willpower. Weight is an extremely intricate problem with handfuls if not hundreds of contributing elements. Various hereditary factors are related to stoutness, and different ailments, like hypothyroidism, PCOS, and gloom, can build your gamble of weight gain. Your body likewise has various chemicals and natural pathways that should manage body weight. These will quite often be useless in individuals with corpulence, making it a lot harder to get more fit and keep it off. For instance, being impervious to the chemical leptin is a significant reason for heftiness. The leptin signal should let your cerebrum know that it has sufficient fat put away. However, assuming you're impervious to leptin, your cerebrum feels that you're starving. Attempting to resolve and deliberately eating less notwithstanding the leptin-driven starvation signal is inconceivably troublesome. This doesn't imply that individuals ought to surrender and acknowledge their hereditary destiny. Getting in shape is as yet conceivable — it's only a lot harder for certain individuals. Heftiness is an extremely intricate problem. Numerous hereditary, organic, and ecological elements influence body weight. Therefore, losing weight isn't just about determination.

MYTH: Eat less, move more

Muscle versus fat is essentially putting away energy.

To lose fat, you want to consume a bigger number of calories than you take in. Therefore, it seems reasonable that eating less and moving more would result in weight loss. While this exhortation works in principle, particularly if you make a long-lasting way of life change, it's a terrible suggestion for those with a serious weight issue. A great many people who heed this guidance wind up recovering any shed pounds because of physiological and biochemical elements. A significant and supported real impact in context and conduct is expected to get thinner with diet and exercise. Limiting your food intake won't help you get more actual work. Training somebody with heftiness to just eat less and move more resembles advising somebody with melancholy to encourage or somebody with liquor abuse to drink less. Advising individuals with weight issues to simply eat less and move more is inadequate guidance that seldom works in the long run.

MYTH: Carbs make you fat

Low-carb diets can help weight reduction. As a rule, this happens even without cognizant calorie limitation. However long you keep carb consumption low and protein admission high, you'll get thinner. All things considered, this doesn't imply that carbs cause weight gain. While the heftiness pandemic began around 1980, people have been eating carbs for quite a while. Entire food sources that are high in carbs are exceptionally sound. Then again, refined carbs like refined grains and sugar are certainly connected to weight gain. Low-carb counts of calories are exceptionally viable for weight reduction. In any case, carbs are not what causes weight in any case. Entire, single-fixing carb-based food sources are unquestionably solid.

MYTH: Fantasy? Scale back carbs to weight loss

Straight forward and complex. Basic carbs found in food varieties like treats and candy need nutrients, minerals, and fiber. Limiting these desserts is a fantastic way to improve your diet and possibly lose weight. Food varieties with complex carbs like entire wheat bread, beans, and natural products, have loads of supplements that are great for you. Scale back straightforward carbs however, keep complex carbs on the menu.

MYTH: Fats make you fat

Fat gives around 9 calories for each gram, contrasted and just 4 calories for every gram of carbs or protein. Fat is very calorie-thick and typical in low-quality foods. However, as long as your calorie admission is inside a sound reach, fat doesn't make you fat.

MYTH: Fast food is continuously stuffing

Not all inexpensive food is undesirable. Given individuals' expanded well-being awareness, many cheap food chains have begun offering better choices. Some, for example, Chipotle, even spotlight solely on serving quality food varieties. It's possible to get something somewhat solid at most eateries. Most modest drive-thru eateries frequently give better options in contrast to their fundamental contributions. These food varieties may not fulfill the requests of every health-cognizant individual, however, they're as yet a fair decision on the off chance that you don't have the opportunity or energy to prepare a good feast. Cheap food doesn't need to be undesirable or swell.

Most cheap food chains offer a few better options in contrast to their principal contributions.

Too old to diet, excessively old to gain muscle: This is wrong. I set up these 2 since the two of them fall under the misrepresentation old enough. Eating less and practicing more, as long as you don't mishandle the cycles, works for all ages. Concentrate on showing long-term olds in a nursing home additional muscle with legitimate activity. Individuals from 16 to 85 get thinner and sound. Doing such under clinical watch might be vital, however, it is possible. What's more, coincidentally, digestion doesn't dial back with age-you do. Get off the lounge chair and do stuff. The more you do, the simpler it is to do.

MYTH: Weight reduction counts calories work

The weight reduction industry believes that you should accept that diets work. Notwithstanding, concentrate on showing that counting calories seldom works in the long haul. Prominently, 85% of calorie counters wind up restoring the load soon. Also, individuals who diet are probably going to put on weight from here on out.

In this way, consuming fewer calories is a reliable indicator of future weight gain, not misfortune. Truly you likely shouldn't move toward weight reduction with an eating fewer carbs mentality. All things considered, make it an objective to change your way of life forever and become a better, more joyful, and fitter individual. If you figure out how to expand your action levels, eat better, and rest better, you ought to shed pounds as a characteristic secondary effect.

MYTH: Eating fewer carbs presumably won't work in the long run

Regardless of what the weight reduction industry would have you accept, slimming down typically doesn't work. It's smarter to change your way of life than to bounce from one eating routine to another in the desire to get in shape. Heftiness is connected to a few persistent illnesses, like sort 2 diabetes. In any case, many individuals with stoutness are metabolically sound, while many dainty individuals are not.

MYTH: Diet food sources can assist you to lose weight

A great deal of low-quality food is promoted as solid. Models incorporate low-fat, sans-fat, and handled-without-gluten food sources, as well as high-sugar refreshments. You ought to have one or two serious misgivings of any well-being claims on food bundling, particularly on handled things. These names normally exist to beguile not illuminate. Some unhealthy food advertisers will urge you to purchase their swelling low-quality food. Truth be told, if the bundling of food lets you know that it's solid, there's an opportunity it's the specific inverse. Periodically, items advertised as diet food sources are unhealthy foods in camouflage, as they're vigorously handled and may hold onto stowed-away fixings.

If you're attempting to get thinner, you might have heard a great deal of similar fantasies. You might have even trusted some of them, as they're difficult to stay away from in Western culture. Outstandingly, a large portion of these legends are bogus All things being equal, the connection between food, your body, and your weight is extremely complicated. Assuming that you're keen on weight reduction, have a go at finding out about the proof-based transformations you can make to your eating regimen and way of life.

MYTH: If the name says "no-fat" or "low-fat," you can eat all you need and not put on weight

Some low-fat or no-fat food varieties have added sugar, starch, or salt to compensate for the decrease in fat. These "wonder" food sources frequently have as many calories, or more, than the customary variant.

Check the nourishment mark to perceive the number of calories that are in a serving. Make certain to check the serving size as well.

MYTH: Skipping breakfast makes you put on weight

Truth: Having a sound breakfast can assist you with dealing with your cravings later in the day and assist you with saying "Not this time" to unfortunate tidbits. No logical investigations have shown that avoiding the morning feast drives straightforwardly to weight gain.

If you are not eager first thing, pay attention to your body. At the point when you are prepared to eat, make a sound choice like cereal with new berries.

MYTH: Eating around the evening time will make you put on weight

Individuals who eat late around the evening time will generally gain additional weight. One potential explanation is that late-night eaters will generally pick unhealthy treats. Certain individuals who nibble after supper don't rest soundly, which can prompt unfortunate desires the following day.

If you are eager after supper, restrict yourself to solid bites like low-fat yogurt or child carrots.

MYTH: You can't be overweight and healthy

Certain individuals are overweight with a sound pulse, cholesterol, and glucose levels. For the vast majority, an overabundance of weight expands the gamble for coronary illness and diabetes. The more you are overweight, the more your gamble of creating infection increases.

MYTH: Fasting can assist you in losing weight

Truly fasting isn't solid assuming you go hungry the entire day and cap it off with an immense feast that replaces every one of the calories you skirted before. In contrast with individuals who lose fat by eating fewer calories, individuals who quickly lose more muscle than fat.

Take a gander at your day-to-day diet for void calories you can remove, like refined grains and sweet beverages. Try not to remove feasts, particularly without a specialist's oversight.

MYTH: You need to lay out humble objectives to shed pounds

In principle, it's a good idea that on the off chance that you put forth aggressive objectives and don't contact them, you could surrender. Nonetheless, certain individuals lose more weight when they put forth objectives that make them propel themselves.

No two individuals are something very similar. It's possible that what works for someone else won't for you. Shedding pounds is a cycle. Be prepared to alter your arrangement as you find what works and doesn't work for you.

20. Slow weight reduction is the best way to get more fit and keep it off:

While the facts confirm that many individuals who lose a great deal of weight in a brief time frame restore everything, this isn't valid for everybody. Certain individuals who are overweight are more fruitful when they get thinner rapidly, for example, going from 300 to 250 pounds (135 to 112 kilograms) in under a year.

Slow weight loss is probably not going to be your main option. Simply be mindful to keep away from craze counts calories that guarantee ridiculous outcomes, they may not be protected. If you are keen on an eating routine that supports quicker weight reduction, make certain to work with your medical care supplier to ensure you are getting every one of the supplements you want.

MYTH: Exercise alone is the answer to weight loss

This isn't accurate. The best method for getting in shape is to lessen the quantity of calories we eat and drink. Exercise can uphold weight reduction when we consume less calories. Weight reduction is still up in the air to the harmony between the calories you consume and the calories you use. While practice is significant for general well-being and can uphold weight reduction, dietary decisions, and calorie consumption assume a more significant part in accomplishing and keeping a solid weight. Research shows that diet assumes a more critical part in weight reduction than exercise alone. It's feasible to work out consistently nevertheless not get more fit if your caloric intake surpasses the calories consumed during exercise. In this way, an exhaustive way to deal with weight reduction ought to incorporate both a decent eating regimen and normal active work.

While practice is an important part of a sound way of life and has various advantages, its effect on weight reduction can at times be misjudged. Several reasons for this include the ones listed below:

1. **Caloric Irregularity:** Exercise consumes calories, yet the quantity of calories consumed in exercise can some of the time be lower than anticipated. For example, a serious exercise could consume two or three hundred calories, yet a solitary fatty dinner could without much of a stretch offset that work. This highlights the significance of being aware of your eating regimen too.

2. **Craving Guideline**: Taking part in exercise can once in a while prompt an expansion in hunger, making a few people consume a bigger number of calories than they consumed during their exercise. This

peculiarity can subvert weight reduction endeavors if is not overseen as expected.

3. **Metabolic Variation:** When you lessen your caloric admission for weight reduction, your body might answer by diminishing its metabolic rate. In this present circumstance, exercise can assist with alleviating the log jam in digestion, however, it cannot completely balance it.

4. **Diet Quality:** The nature of your eating routine fundamentally affects weight reduction. A fair eating routine that gives fundamental supplements and controls segment sizes is fundamental. Depending exclusively on practice without focusing on the dietary substance of your feasts can prevent progress.

5. **Stationary Way of Life:** For certain individuals, depending exclusively on exercise can prompt an inactive way of life beyond their exercise meetings. Being stationary for a large portion of the day checks the advantages of activity and might have negative well-being impacts.

6. **Individual Variety:** Individuals' bodies answer distinctively to exercise and dietary changes. Hereditary qualities, hormonal elements, and metabolic contrasts can

impact how viable activity is for weight reduction on a singular premise.

While it is essential for generally speaking well-being and has different advantages past weight reduction, it is not the sole factor that decides effective weight. A far-reaching way to deal with weight reduction includes a fair diet, portion control, normal physical activity, and care about caloric intake. The practicing of these variables results in practical and viable weight reduction.

Chapter 4
Designing Your Plate for Weight Loss

The Plate method is an aid for getting a meal that can assist you with weight reduction. The Plate method can assist with weight reduction and adjusted eating. It is not difficult to use. Most dinners can include a lot of vegetables. They also have protein and a high-fiber starch. You could add low-fat dairy, high fat, and organic products to the dinner. A morning meal bowl with eggs, Asian fish salad, skillet-burned salmon, and spaghetti with meat sauce are four instances of meals given the Plate Technique.

Making a meal for weight reduction is simple. Furthermore, you can get a fair dinner without being a nutritionist. The main device you want is a plate.

How may you do this? The Plate Strategy can help.

You can relax. The Plate method is adaptable. It can go with a variety of eating habits and food preferences. What's more, as the Dietary Rules for Americans call attention to, little changes can amount to durable outcomes. Continue to peruse to gain proficiency with the advantages of the Plate method. You can learn how to make use of it. There is likewise an example of breakfast, lunch, and supper in light of the Plate method.

Benefit of the Plate method

Using the Plate method can keep you from eating a lot without acknowledging it. It can likewise assist you with the following.

- Make a good dinner without being a nutritionist.
- Adhere to your feast plan without troublesome weight or estimating food sources.
- Give you more fiber and protein so feasts are really filling and you are not ravenous soon thereafter.

Furthermore, the Plate method can assist you with building a nutritious dinner without being a specialist. At the point when you adhere to the rules beneath, your dinner will have savvy measures of protein, solid fat, and high-fiber sugars.

Parts of the Plate

In the first place, you need a plate. A standard supper plate has a measurement of 10 to 12 inches, however, it is likewise suggested to use a plate with a 9-inch width.

You don't have to purchase another arrangement of dishes if your plates are bigger. These are a few choices.

- Use a huge treat plate all things considered.
- Use your ordinary supper plate, yet don't put food around the edge.
- Avoid worrying about it as much as you can.

Since you have your plate, this goes on it.

- Fill around 50% of your plate with Non-starchy vegetables.
- One-fourth of your plate with lean protein.
- One-fourth of your plate with sound sugars.
- Water or another 0-calorie drink can go with your dinner.

Non-starchy Vegetables

Non-starchy vegetables should cover half of your plate. Eat them raw or set them up just. Cook, barbecue, steam, or microwave them as opposed to searing them to limit fat. Stay away from a lot of dressing, cooking fats like margarine or oil, and velvety sauces. Non-starchy vegetables include these:

- Salad and different greens, for example, lettuces, spinach, collard greens, spring blend, kale, and mustard greens
- Tomatoes, eggplant, chime peppers, zucchini.
- Cucumbers, mushrooms, carrots, celery
- Broccoli, cauliflower, cabbage, bok choy, Artichokes, asparagus, green beans, onions.

Lean Protein

Split the other portion of your plate into equal parts to make quarters. Lean protein goes in one quarter. You could pick any of these:

Thin chicken, lean ground turkey, Salmon, trout, fish, shrimp, and other fish and shellfish

Egg substitute, egg, or egg whites, Curds, Tofu, beans, lentils, veggie burger

Try to search for less-processed food varieties that are low in undesirable fats. Bacon processed meat, and greasy red meat are not lean proteins.

Healthy Carbohydrates

The last quarter of your plate has a sound Carbohydrate. What is a "healthy" Carbohydrate? They are less handled. They are high in fiber and different supplements. They are low in added sugars. They are connected to bring down body weight.

They include the following:

- Whole grains, like grain, earthy colored rice, or quinoa.
- Whole wheat pasta or bread, like cut bread, pita, or English biscuit
- Whole grain breakfast cereal or oats, Potatoes, oak seed squash, yam, corn, or peas.

- Likewise with non-bland vegetables, keeping these low in sugar or undesirable fat is ideal. For instance, pick unsweetened grains, and breaking point greasy or velvety dishes like pureed potatoes, French fries, and fettuccine Alfredo.

Diary and fruit Items

The Dietary Rules for Americans recommend utilizing MyPlate.gov from the US Branch of Agribusiness (USDA). These dinners may likewise include:

A decreased-fat dairy item, like skim milk, low-fat cheddar, or non-fat plain yogurt.

A serving of new natural products, like a little apple, 2 tangerines, 1/2 cup of grapes, or 1 cup of strawberries.

Some sound fat, for example, avocado, nuts, or nut margarine, or 1 to 2 teaspoons of olive oil utilized in cooking or salad dressing.

Dairy items add calcium and protein. The new fruit has fiber and cell reinforcements. Also, solid fats assist with lessening hunger and forestalling glucose spikes.

Test Plate meals

What does a Plate method or MyPlate.gov meal seem to be? Here are a few models.

Test Plate Dinner 1: Breakfast Bowl

This bowl has around 400 calories.

- Hard-bubbled or other cooked egg which contains Protein.
- Salad with ½ cup of sliced tomatoes, ¼ slashed cucumber, 1 tablespoon of diced onion, 1 teaspoon of olive oil, and balsamic vinegar. They are Non-starchy vegetables, Organic products, and Solid fat.
- 1.5 ounces of low-fat feta cheddar.

Test Plate Dinner 2: Asian Fish Salad

This is a simple dinner that is not difficult to prepare in a lunch sack. You can make the fish salad the prior night and let the flavors blend.

- Asian fish salad with 3 ounces of canned fish, 3 tablespoons of plain yogurt, ¼ cup of diced apple, 2 tablespoons of slashed celery, diced onion, cleaved cilantro, ¼ cup of hacked tomato, run every one of low-sodium soy sauce, rice wine vinegar, dark pepper, stew glue, and 2 teaspoons of sesame oil. They contain Protein, Solid fat, fruits, Non-starchy vegetables, and Low-fat dairy.

- A bed of greens like arugula it's a
  Non-starchy vegetable
- 1 cup of whole wheat bread. High-fiber
  sugar and 1 tangerine.

Test Plate Feast 3: Skillet Singed Salmon Supper with Simmered Broccoli

This supper has under 500 calories. You can trade any protein, like chicken or tofu, for salmon.

- 3 ounces of salmon, skillet signed with
  cooking spray. Contains Protein and solid
  fat.
- Simmered broccoli with 1 teaspoon of olive
  oil, finished off with 1 ounce of low-fat blue
  or cheddar. Contains Non-starchy
  vegetables, Solid fat, and reduced-fat dairy.
- ⅓ cup of cooked brown-colored rice.
  High-fiber sugar
- ½ cup of blueberries. Fruit.

Test Plate Feast 4 - Spaghetti Supper

Youngsters and grown-ups the same can adore the Plate Strategy! Here is a fair spaghetti supper. You can add a lettuce-based side plate of mixed greens if you like.

- ½ cup of cooked entire wheat spaghetti
  which is High-fiber carb.
- Pureed tomatoes with ½ cup of
  tomato-based pasta sauce (search for a brand

without any than 3 grams of added sugar), 3 ounces of lean turkey with Italian flavoring, and ½ cup of cooked vegetables, for example, cut mushrooms or sliced ringer pepper. Which contains Protein and non-starchy vegetables.

- 1 ounce of reduced-fat parmesan cheddar. Decreased fat dairy
- 1 cup of new cut natural product, ½ ounce of almonds or different nuts. Which contains Fruit and Healthy fat.

The 50/50 Plate method for Weight reduction

The objective of the 50/50 plate is to bring down the calorie thickness of your dinner. Fill one portion of your plate with a non-starchy vegetable and the opposite side of your plate with negligibly processed starches.

By doing this, you are enormously bringing down the calories of your dinner without losing the food volume. For this reason, the 50/50 plate is so successful because you are not left feeling hungry after a feast.

For instance, while eating a plate of heavenly lentil Bolognese and pasta you would serve yourself the pasta on one side and broccoli on the other. You need to see a reasonable line down the center of your plate so you realize without a doubt that you made the 50/50 plate equivalent.

So the greatest change in calories of a food is how much water and fiber is in it. Since when you eliminate water you make the food a more focused calorie source. To this end, any sort of food handling makes food varieties more calorie thick.

These two plates are comparable in calories however you'd feel fairly full on the grapes and jeer the raisins in no time flat. Plant food sources in their normal structure impeccably defend us from gorging, because we genuinely battle to eat such a large number of calories.

If you're trying to get into a calorie shortage for weight reduction, you don't have to know your calories in or your calories out, you simply have to deal with lessening your calories intake at this point! The 50/50 plate is the least demanding and best approach to doing precisely that.

Real-life Example.

Think about it concerning cash. You want to set aside cash, so you begin spending $50 less every week. You don't have to know the current balance in your bank yet, rather, simply reduce how much your ongoing starting point is. If you know that the vast majority of your spending goes towards eating out 5 times each week, as opposed to working out the number of meals you need to remove seven days to get to $50 you could quit eating out during the week.

The 50/50 plate is a demonstrated method for reducing your general calories without counting. They are more charming and long-lasting.

Portion Control

Portion control means choosing an appropriate amount of a particular food. Portion control assists you with getting the advantages of the supplements in the food without overeating. Portion control is essential because it helps you to digest food more easily, reach or keep a sound weight, retain energy throughout the day, and control sugar levels.

Why is portion control important?

In essential terms, your body requires a specific measure of calories to work and endure every day. Those are determined by your age, current weight, and everyday activity level and differ from one individual to another. A normal lady requires roughly 2000 calories each day to keep up with her weight, and 1500 calories each day to lose one pound of weight each week. A normal man, then again, requires around 2,500 calories each day to keep up with his weight, and 2000 to lose one pound of weight each week.

That is where portion control comes in. If you're eating a larger number of calories than your body needs, your body will take those additional calories and store them as fat. You will store more fat if you eat more calories than you need to. Along these lines, to decrease those additional calories being put away as fat, we can use portion control to ensure we are eating what our body requires.

The justification for why this is so hard for the vast majority of us to do is we are continually given bigger parts than we want. This makes us eat more without acknowledging we've over-eaten, causing weight gain.

10 Tips to Quantify and Control Portion Sizes

People will generally eat practically all of what they serve themselves. Therefore, controlling Portion sizes can help forestall indulging. The following are 10 hints to gauge and control portion sizes both at home and in a hurry.

1. Use More modest Dinnerware

Proof recommends that sizes of plates, spoons, and glasses can unknowingly impact how much food somebody eats. For instance, using larger plates can cause food to seem more modest, frequently prompting indulgence. individuals using an large bowl ate 77% more pasta than those using a medium-sized bowl. Nourishing specialists served themselves 31% more frozen yogurt when given bigger dishes and 14.5% more when given bigger serving spoons. Curiously, the vast majority who ate more because of huge dishes were ignorant about the adjustment of piece size. In this manner, trading your typical plate, bowl, or serving spoon for a more modest option can decrease the aiding of food and forestall overeating. The vast majority feel similarly as full having eaten from a more modest dish than from an enormous one.

Essentially using more modest dishes or glasses can bring down how much food or drink you consume. Furthermore, individuals will generally feel similarly fulfilled.

2. Using Your Plate as a Part Guide

Try using your plate or bowl as a portion control guide if estimating or overeating food doesn't appeal to you. This can assist you with deciding the ideal macronutrient proportion for an even feast. A harsh aide for every dinner is:

Vegetables or salad: A portion of a plate

Protein: A quarter of a plate, with meat, poultry, fish, eggs, dairy, tofu, and beans.

Complex carbs: Quarter of a plate such as whole grains and vegetables

High-fat food sources: A portion of a tablespoon (7 grams). Including cheese, oils, and butter.

Don't forget that this is just a rough guide, as people have different dietary necessities. For instance, the people who are all the more truly dynamic frequently require more food. As vegetables and salad are normally low in calories but high in fiber and different supplements, topping off on these may assist you with trying not to gorge on calorie-thick food varieties. On the off chance that you need additional direction, a few producers sell segment control plates. Involving a plate as an aide for segment control can assist you with checking complete food consumption. You can separate your plate into areas in light of various nutrition types.

3. Using Your Hands as a Serving Direction

One more method for checking suitable part size with practically no estimating devices is by basically using your hands.

As your hands generally compare to your body size, huge people who require more food ordinarily have greater hands.

A rough aide for every dinner is:

- High-protein food sources: A palm-sized serving for ladies and two palm-sized portions for men like meat, fish, poultry, and beans.
- Vegetables and mixed greens: A clenched hand-measured portion for ladies and two clenched hand-measured portions for men

- High-carb food sources: One measured hand portion for ladies and two for men like whole grains and vegetables.
- High-fat food varieties: One thumb-sized portion for ladies and two for men like spread, oils, and nuts.

Your Hands can be a useful aide for portion sizes. Different nutrition types compare to different shapes and portions of your hands.

4. Request for a Half portion While Eating Out

Restaurants are infamous for serving enormous portions. Overall, around 2.5 times bigger than standard serving sizes and up to an incredible multiple times bigger. If you are eating out, you can continuously request a half-piece or a kids' dish. This will save you a great deal of calories and assist with forestalling gorging. On the other hand, you could impart a feast to somebody or request a starter and side rather than a primary dish. Different tips incorporate requesting a side plate of mixed greens or vegetables, requesting sauces and dressings to be served independently, and staying away from buffet-style, all-you-can-eat cafés where it's exceptionally simple to indulge. Café portions will generally be no less than two times the size of a standard part. Forestall indulges by requesting a half part, requesting a starter rather than a principal dish, and staying away from buffet-style eateries.

5. Begin All Dinners With a Glass of Water

Drinking a glass of water as long as 30 minutes before dinner will normally help segment control. Topping off on water will cause you to feel less eager. Being all around hydrated likewise assists you with recognizing cravings and thirst. One concentrate in moderately aged and more seasoned grown-ups saw that drinking 17 ounces (500 ml) of water before every dinner brought about a 44% more noteworthy decrease in weight north of 12 weeks, undoubtedly because of diminished food consumption. Likewise, when overweight and fat more seasoned grown-ups drank 17 ounces (500 ml) of water 30 minutes before dinner, and they polished off 13% fewer calories without attempting to roll out any improvements.

Typical weight men drinking a comparable measure of water preceding a dinner brought about more noteworthy sensations of totality and diminished food consumption. Subsequently, having a glass of water before every feast can assist with forestalling indulging and help portion control. Drinking a glass of water as long as 30 minutes before a meal can normally bring about a reduction in food consumption and more prominent sensations of totality.

6. Take It Slowly

Eating rapidly makes you less mindful of getting full and in this way improves your probability of overeating. As your mind can require about 20 minutes to make sure that you are full after eating, dialing back can lessen your all-out intake. For instance, one concentrated in solid ladies noticed that eating gradually prompted more noteworthy sensations of completion and a decline in food consumption contrasted with What's more, the ones who ate gradually would in general partake in their dinner more Furthermore, eating in a hurry or while occupied or staring at the television helps your probability of gorging. Therefore, zeroing in on your dinner and declining to rush expands the possibility you'll appreciate it and control your piece sizes. Taking more modest chomps and biting each significant piece somewhere around five or multiple times before gulping. Plunking down to feasts with no interruptions and eating gradually will manage segment control and decrease your probability of indulging.

7. Try not to consume food straight from the container.

Enormous size bundles or food served from huge holders energizes overeating and less attention to suitable part measures. This is particularly valid for snacks. Individuals will generally eat more out of enormous bundles than little ones paying little mind to food taste or quality. For instance, individuals ate 129% more confections when served from a huge container than a little one. In another review, members consumed over 180 fewer grams of snacks each week when given 100-gram nibble packs than when given snacks in standard-sized bundles. As opposed to eating snacks from the first bundling, empty them into a little bowl to prevent eating an excess. A similar applies to the mass portion of family meals. As opposed to serving food straightforwardly from the oven, re-portion it onto plates before serving. Doing so will help forestall stuffing your plate and deter returning for seconds. Eating food from bigger bundles or compartments energizes expanded admission. Attempt re-distributing snacks into individual partitions and serving family dinners from plates to forestall indulging.

8. Know about Reasonable Serving Size

Research shows that we can't necessarily depend on our judgement of suitable piece size. This is because many variables influence portion control. Nonetheless, it might assist with putting resources into a scale or measuring cup to weigh food and accurately survey your intake. Studying food names likewise expands attention to appropriate portions. It is suggested serving sizes for generally eaten food sources can assist you with directing your admission.

Here are a few examples:

- **Cooked Rice or pasta:** 1/2 cup (75 and 100 grams, respectively).
- **Vegetables also, salad:** 1-2 cups (150-300 grams).
- **Breakfast oat:** 1 cup (40 grams).
- **Cooked beans:** 1/2 cup (90 grams).
- **Nut spread:** 2 tablespoons (16 grams) Cooked meats: 3 ounces (85 grams).

You don't necessarily need to quantify your dinners. Be that as it may, doing so might be useful for a brief period to foster a consciousness of what a proper piece size resembles. Sooner or later, you should not have to quantify everything. Using measuring equipment can assist with expanding consciousness of part measures and accurately evaluating how much food is ordinarily eaten.

9. Using a Food Diary

Individuals are frequently amazed at how much food they eat. For instance, one study found that 21% of people who ate more because their serving bowls were bigger denied doing so. Recording all food and drink admissions can build familiarity with the kind and measure of food sources you're polishing off. In weight reduction studies, the people who kept a food journal would in general lose more weight by and large. This probably happened because they turned out to be more mindful of what they ate including their unfortunate decisions and changed their eating routine as needed. Writing down your absolute calorie admission can expand attention to what you consume. This can spur you to pursue better decisions and decrease your possibility of overeating.

10. Drink From a Tall Straight Glass

You can have liquor or a soda with your feast, yet hold it to one glass and enjoy it slowly. individuals drank increasingly slowly from glasses that were straight-edged, contrasted with outward-inclined. limit your intake of sweet drinks and only one 12-ounce container of standard soft drink contains 10 teaspoons of sugar, an entire four teaspoons more than what's recommended for every day for women, or an additional teaspoon for men. Adult women ought to restrict themselves to one beverage and grown-up men two beverages (12 ounces of lager; 5 ounces of wine) or less in a day.

Unwanted weight gain might begin with huge portion sizes. In any case, there are numerous viable advances you can take to control portions. These basic changes have demonstrated fruitful in lessening portions without settling on taste or sensations of completion. For instance, measuring your food, using more modest dishes, drinking water before feasting, and eating slowly can all lessen your risk of overeating. Toward the day's end, portion control is a convenient solution that works to your satisfaction.

Chapter 5
Eating for Specific Goals

Every person may have different goals when it comes to their health and body composition, so no one diet works for everyone. Setting specific goals for your diet is crucial for success, whether you want to manage a particular health condition, gain muscle, lose weight, or improve athletic performance. Here is a thorough guide to choosing foods to achieve particular objectives while dieting.

Eating for Weight Loss

If you want to lose weight, concentrate on establishing a calorie deficit by taking in fewer calories than your body expends. Include nutrient-dense foods like fresh produce, whole grains, lean proteins, and healthy fats in your diet.

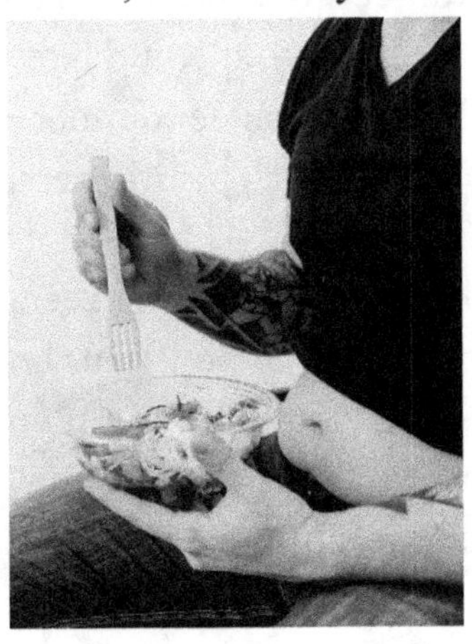

Consider tracking your intake with apps or food journals, and be aware of portion sizes. Steer clear of processed foods with lots of calories and sugar. The effective methods to shed pounds include the following:

1. Eat protein, fat, and vegetables: Aims to include various food varieties at every meal. To adjust your plate, your dinners ought to include protein, fat, vegetables, and complex carbs.

2. Move your body: The Active Work Rules for Americans suggest consolidating cardio exercises with powerlifting for ideal well-being. Cardio exercises include things like strolling, running, running, cycling, or swimming.

3. Eat more fiber: Fiber moves gradually through the intestinal system and can assist you with feeling fuller for longer to help weight reduction. It could likewise settle sugar levels, advance routineness, and safeguard against specific persistent circumstances.

4. Eat mindfully: Having a decent comprehension of how your body responds to food and eating can assist you with ensuring you're not overeating. This is known as mindful eating. It can include eating all the more leisurely, figuring out

how to perceive when you're eager versus while you're longing for nourishment for profound reasons, cooking brilliant food varieties with different surfaces to drag out and partake in your dinners

5. Remain hydrated: Drinking a lot of water can assist with advancing weight reduction by decreasing your food consumption, particularly if you hydrate before dinner. It could likewise work by expanding fat consumption, which can assist with upgrading long-haul weight reduction.

Eating for Muscle Gain

The muscle gain object is usually partaken by bodybuilders. Bodybuilding is tied in with looking strong and lean. To assist you with arriving at this goal, you need to eat nutrient-rich food varieties with bunches of protein while restricting alcohol and sweet or southern-style foods. Working out centers around building your body's muscles through weight lifting and nourishment.

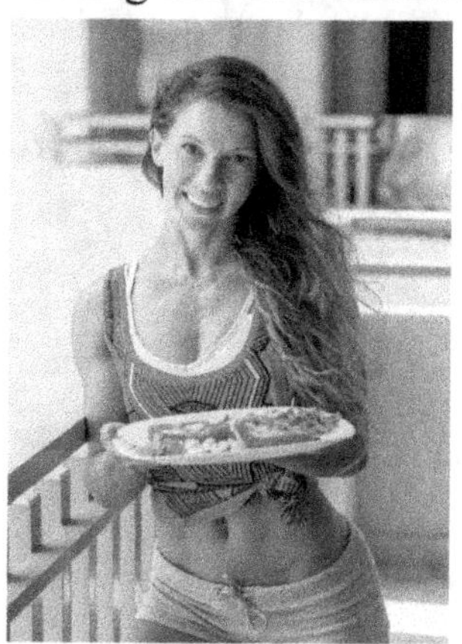

To maximize your outcomes from the gym, you pay attention to your diet, as eating some unacceptable food varieties can hinder your bodybuilding goals. The goal for competitive bodybuilders is to increase bulk in the building stage and reduce body fat in the cutting stage. Therefore, you consume a larger number of calories in the building stage than in the cutting stage.

How many calories do you Need?

During your building stage, you should increase your calorie intake by around 15%. For instance, if your support calories are 3,000 every day, you should eat 3,450 calories each day (3,000 x 0.15 = 450) during your building stage You would prefer to consume 15% fewer upkeep calories as you transition from a building to a cutting stage, which would mean eating 2,550 calories daily rather than 3,450. Increase your calories as you put on weight in the building stage and lessen your calories as you lose weight in the cutting stage to proceed with movement.

Protein and carbs contain four calories for every gram (g), and fat contains nine. Recommended intake include:

- 30-35% of your calories from protein
- 55-60% of your calories from carbs
- 15-20% of your calories from fat.

Here is an illustration of the ratio for both a building and cutting stage:

	Building stage	Cutting stage
Calories	3450	2550
Protein (g)	259-302	191-223
Sugars (g).	474-518	351-383
Fat (g)	58-77	43-57

Kind of Foods to Focus on

The food varieties you eat don't have to vary between the building and cutting stage normally, it is the quantity that does.

- Meats, poultry, and fish: Salmon, tilapia, cod, pork tenderloin, venison, chicken breast, ground beef, and sirloin steak.
- Dairy: low-fat milk, cheddar, curds, and Yogurt.
- Grains: Bread, cereal, wafers, oats, quinoa, popcorn, and rice.
- Organic products: Oranges, apples, bananas, grapes, pears, peaches, watermelons, and berries.
- Starchy vegetables: cassava, green lima beans, Potatoes, green peas, and corn.

- Vegetables: green beans, tomatoes, broccoli, spinach, cucumber, zucchini, asparagus, peppers, and mushrooms.
- Seeds and nuts: Almonds, pecans, sunflower seeds, chia seeds, and flax seeds.
- Beans and vegetables: pinto beans, kidney beans, dark beans, and chickpeas.
- oils: avocado, flaxseed, and olive oils.

Food varieties to avoid or Restrict

While you should remember different food varieties in your diet, there are some you should restrict. These include:

- Liquor: Liquor can adversely influence your capacity to assemble muscle and lose fat, particularly if you consume it in overabundance.
- Added sugars: This proposition has a lot of calories however a couple of supplements. Foods with a lot of added sugar include sweets, doughnuts, frozen yogurt, cake, and beverages with added sugar, like pop and sports drinks.
- Pan-fried foods: These may advance aggravation and when devoured in abundance illness. Models incorporate broiled fish, french fries, onion rings, chicken fingers, and cheddar curds.

To build muscle, emphasize protein intake as it provides the building blocks for muscle repair and growth. Include sources such as lean meats, poultry, fish, eggs, dairy products, legumes, and plant-based proteins. Consume complex carbohydrates to fuel your workouts and healthy fats for overall well-being. Additionally, strength training and adequate rest are crucial for muscle development.

Eating for Heart Health

For cardiovascular health, opt for a balanced diet low in saturated and trans fats. Focus on the following foods.

When you add these to food sources rather than salt and fat, you're making a heart-health decision. They add flavor without the bad stuff. Flavors and different food varieties are delightful for heart health.

Fatty fish and fish oil

Fatty fish like salmon, mackerel, sardines, and fish are stacked with omega-3 unsaturated fats, which have been read up broadly for their heart-medical advantages. Omega-3 unsaturated fats from greasy fish might play a defensive part in the gamble of creating coronary illness and marginally lessen the gamble of CVD occasions and arrhythmias. Eating fish for a long time might uphold lower levels of all-out cholesterol, blood fatty oils, fasting glucose, and systolic circulatory strain.

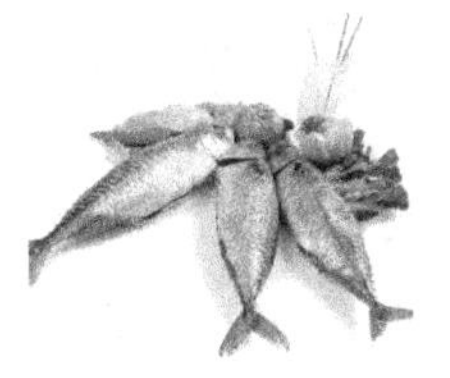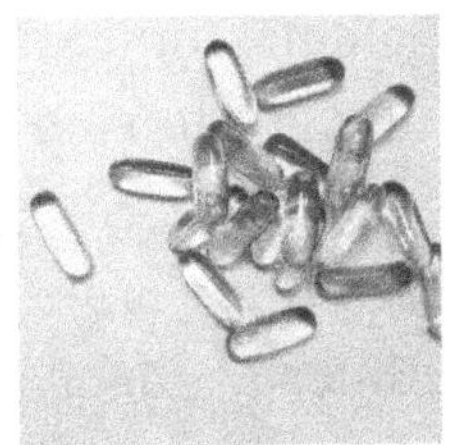

Fish utilization is related to a lower chance of cardiovascular sickness, gloom, and mortality. If you don't eat a lot of fish, fish oil is one more choice for getting your day-to-day portion of omega-3 unsaturated fats.

Leafy green vegetables

Leafy green vegetables like spinach, kale, and collard greens are notable for their abundance of nutrients, minerals, and cell reinforcements. Specifically, they're an extraordinary wellspring of vitamin K, which safeguards your conduits and advances legitimate blood thickening.

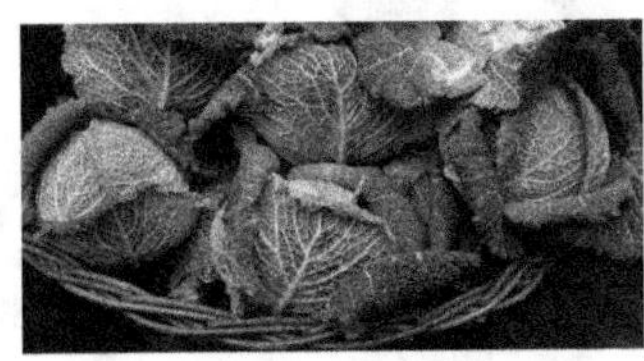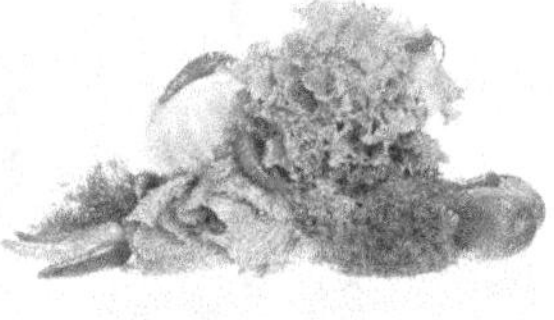

They're likewise high in dietary nitrates, which have been displayed to lessen circulatory strain, decline blood vessel solidness, and work on the capability of cells covering the veins. The American Heart Affiliation (AHA) noticed that an expanded verdant green vegetable admission was related to additional huge advantages to cardiovascular well-being and a lower chance of coronary illness than different leafy foods. Verdant green vegetables are high in vitamin K and nitrates, which can assist with diminishing circulatory strain and work on blood vessel capability. A higher admission of mixed greens is related to a lower chance of coronary illness.

Walnut

Walnuts are an incredible wellspring of fiber and micronutrients like magnesium, copper, and manganese. Research shows that adding a couple of servings of pecans into your eating routine can help safeguard against coronary illness. Proof for cardiovascular illness counteraction is solid for certain assortments of tree nuts, especially pecans.

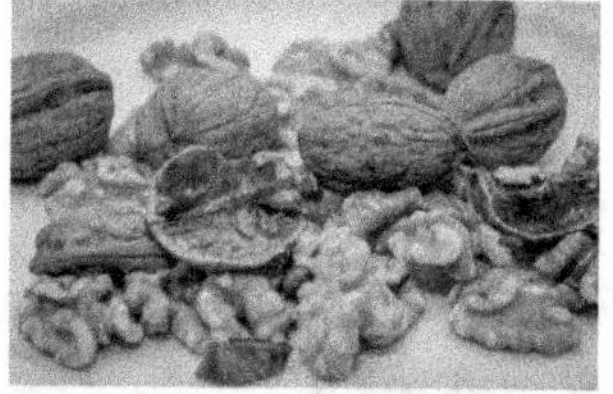

Consuming fewer calories increases with walnuts may decrease LDL (terrible) and complete cholesterol. Strangely, a few examinations likewise found that regularly eating nuts, like walnuts, is related to a lower chance of coronary illness.

Tomatoes

Tomatoes are stacked with lycopene, a characteristic plant shade with strong cell reinforcement properties. Cell reinforcements assist with killing hurtful free revolutionaries, forestalling oxidative harm and aggravation, which can add to coronary illness. Low blood levels of lycopene are connected to an expanded gamble of cardiovascular failure and stroke. Increasing the intake of tomato items and lycopene supplementation decidedly influences blood lipids, pulse, and endothelial capability.

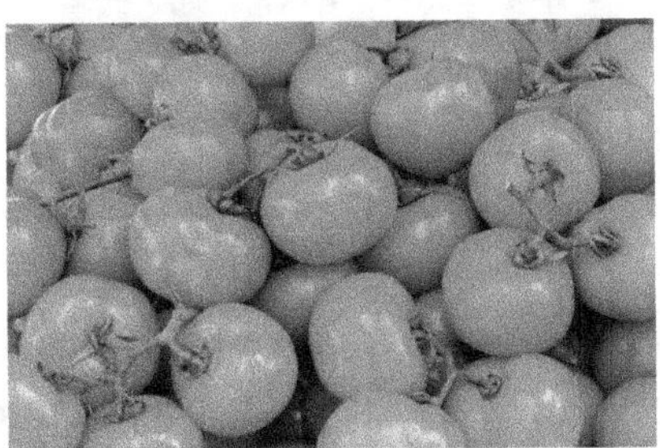

One serving of raw tomatoes, pureed tomatoes, or pureed tomatoes with refined olive oil might bring down blood cholesterol and fatty substances and raise HDL cholesterol. The body retains lycopene better from cooked tomatoes and tomato items than from new tomatoes. Higher HDL (great) cholesterol levels can assist with eliminating an abundance of cholesterol and plaque from the conduits to keep your heart sound and safeguard against coronary illness and stroke.

Beans

Beans contain safe starch, which opposes assimilation and is aged by the useful microorganisms in your stomach. Safe starch might have a sound effect on the stomach and certain individuals from its occupant microbiota.

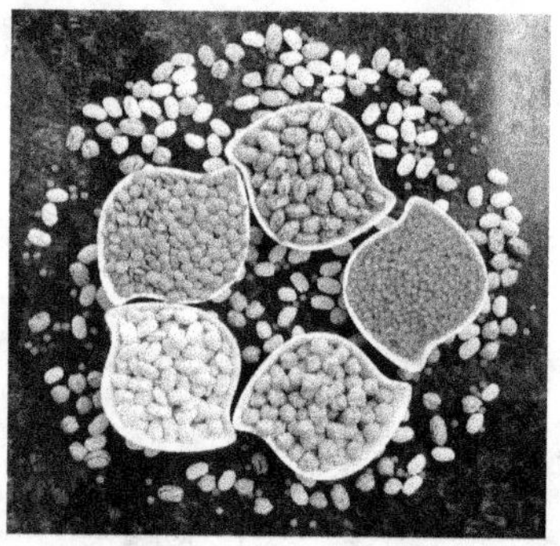

Numerous investigations have likewise found that eating beans can diminish specific gamble factors for coronary illness. In one investigation of 73 adults with raised LDL cholesterol, eating canned beans altogether decreased complete cholesterol and LDL cholesterol. Eating beans and vegetables can decrease LDL cholesterol, improve glycemic control and circulatory strain, and may lessen the gamble of cardiovascular sickness, particularly in individuals with diabetes. Beans are high in safe starch and have been displayed to diminish levels of cholesterol, lower pulse, and improve glycemic control.

Dark chocolate

Dark chocolate is rich in cell reinforcements like flavonoids, which can assist with supporting heart wellbeing. Consuming chocolate with some restraint (under six servings per week) may diminish your risk of heart disease, stroke, and diabetes.

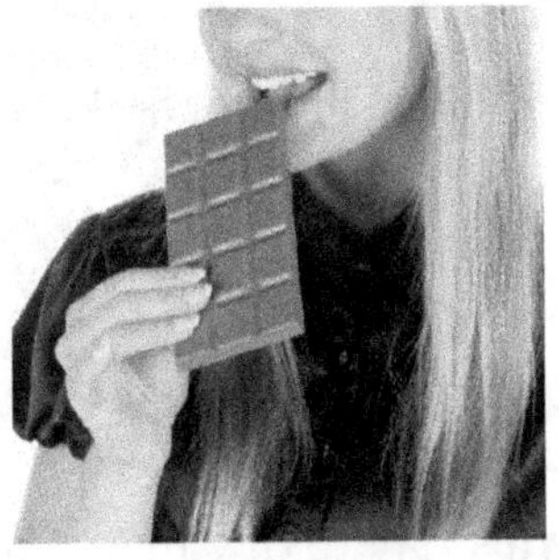

Furthermore, chocolate can be high in sugar and calories, nullifying a significant number of its well-being-advancing properties. Be certain to pick a top-notch dark chocolate with a cocoa content of not less than 70% and moderate your intake to capitalize on its heart-health advantages. Dark chocolate is high in cell reinforcements like flavonoids. It has been related to a lower hazard of creating calcified plaque in the courses and heart disease.

Berries

Strawberries, blueberries, blackberries, and raspberries are jam-loaded with supplements that assume a focal part in heart well-being. Berries are also a rich source of cell defences like anthocyanins, which protect against oxidative stress and irritation that can hasten the progression of coronary disease. Higher anthocyanin intake might raise your gamble of coronary corridor sickness, including respiratory failure and hypertension.

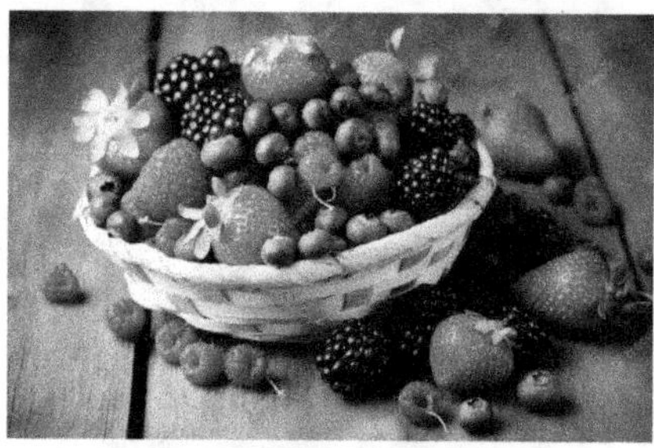

Eating blueberries day to day may likewise work on the capability of cells that line the veins (vascular capability), which assist with controlling pulse and blood thickening. As per a survey of exploration, berry utilization might be a viable mediation for metabolic disorders by lessening oxidative pressure and irritation while working on vascular capability. Berries can be a delightful bite or a scrumptious pastry. Have a go at adding one or two sorts to your eating routine to exploit their medical advantages. Berries are rich in cell reinforcements. Eating them can decrease numerous factors for coronary illness.

Olive oil

Olive oil is loaded with antioxidants, which can free inflammation and decrease the case of persistent sickness. It's additionally rich in monounsaturated unsaturated fats, which many examinations have related to enhancements in heart health.

One review from 2014 implying 7,216 adults at high risk for coronary illness showed that the people who consumed the most olive oil had a 35% lower chance of developing heart problems.

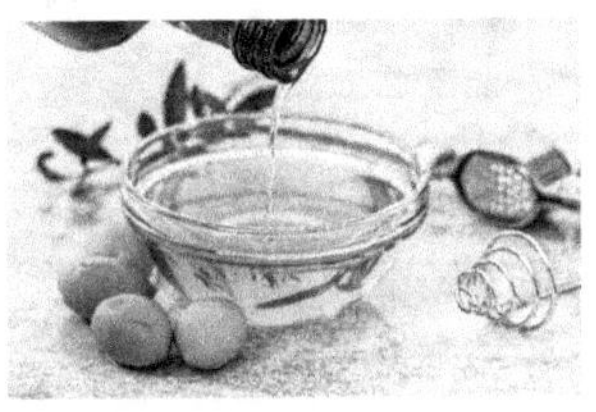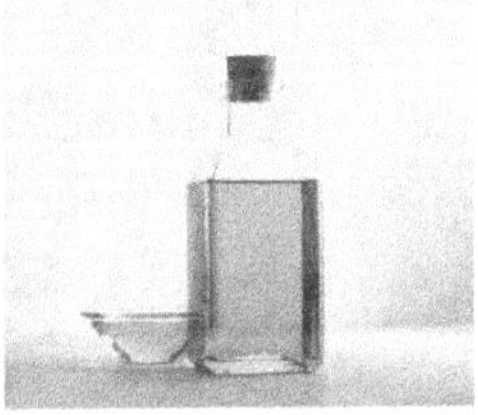

Furthermore, a higher intake of olive oil was related to a 48% lower chance of dying from heart disease. Olive oil is high in oleic corrosive and cell reinforcements and can help forestall and treat hypertension. You can sprinkle olive oil over cooked dishes or add it to vinaigrettes and sauces. Olive oil is high in cancer prevention agents and monounsaturated fats. It has been related to lower blood and heart disease risk.

Almonds

Almonds are unquestionably nutrient-dense, flaunting numerous nutrients and minerals significant to heart health. They're likewise a decent wellspring of heart-solid monounsaturated fats and fiber, two significant supplements that can help safeguard against coronary illness.

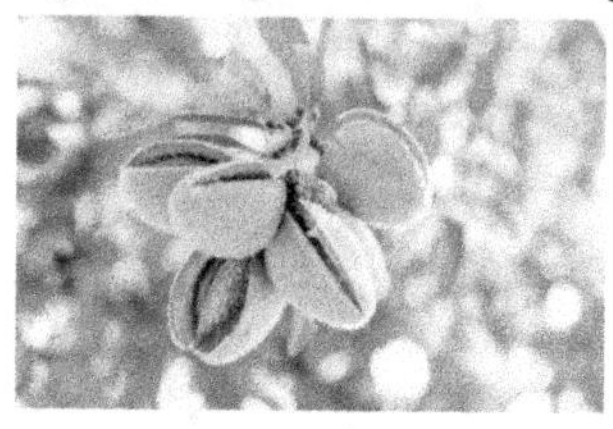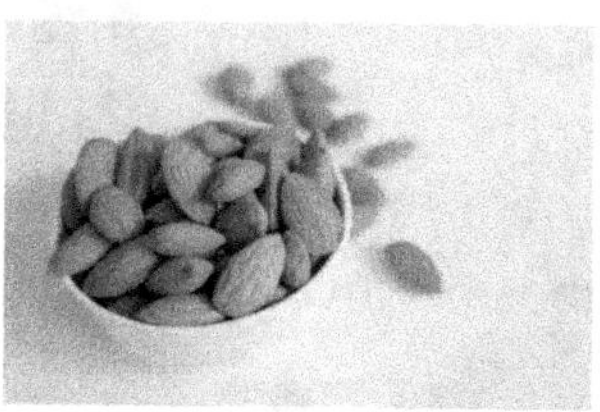

Research recommends that eating almonds can possibly affect your cholesterol levels. One review affecting 48 individuals with elevated cholesterol showed that eating 1.5 ounces (43 grams) of almonds every day for a very long time decreases stomach fat and levels of LDL (terrible) cholesterol, two risk factors for heart disease. Eating almonds is related to more elevated levels of HDL (great) cholesterol, which can assist with lessening plaque development and keep your corridors clear. Remember that while almonds are extremely high in nutrients, they're also high in calories. Measure your bits and moderate your intake if you're attempting to get thinner. Almonds are high in fiber and monounsaturated fats and have been connected to decreases in cholesterol and gut fat.

Garlic

Garlic has powerful restorative properties that might assist with further developing heart wellbeing. This is thanks to the presence of a compound called allicin, which is accepted to make numerous restorative impacts. A meta-investigation of 12 preliminaries noticed that garlic supplements brought down both systolic and diastolic pulses and were as compelling as a typical doctor-prescribed drug at lessening circulatory strain. Garlic can likewise restrain platelet development, which might decrease the risk of blood clots and stroke.

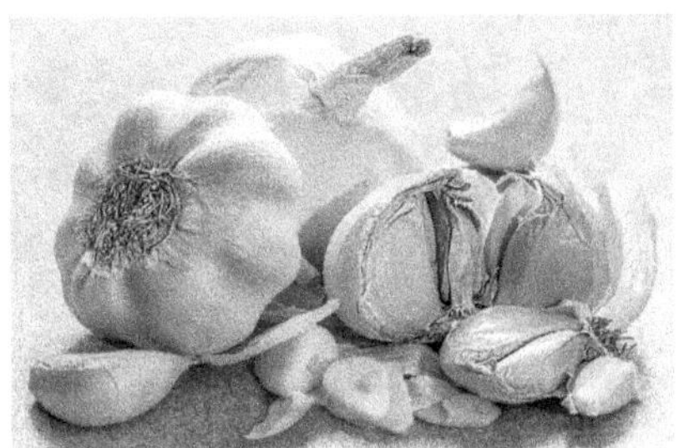

Be certain to consume garlic raw or pound it and allow it to sit for a couple of moments before cooking. This takes into consideration the development of allicin, augmenting its potential medical advantages. Garlic and its parts have been displayed to assist with decreasing blood pressure and cholesterol. They may likewise assist with inhibiting blood clot development.

Eating for Diabetes Management

For people who are seeking a way to manage their diabetes from the type of food they eat, aim for consistent carbohydrate intake throughout the day to regulate blood sugar levels. Choose complex carbohydrates, and fiber-rich foods, and avoid sugary snacks and beverages. Consume healthy fats, and lean proteins, and maintain a balanced diet.

Best foods recommendation for people living with diabetes

1. **Fatty fish:**

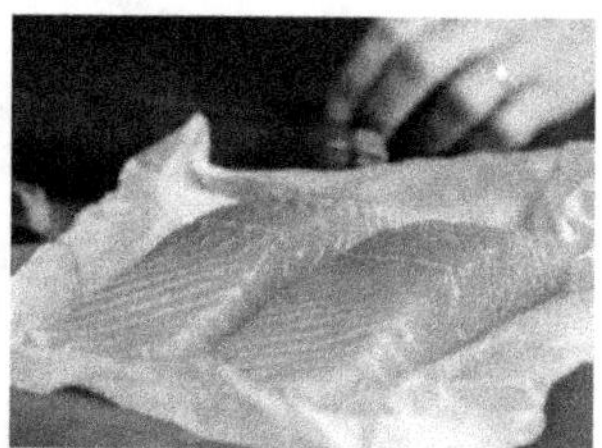

Fatty fish contain omega-3 fats that can assist with reducing inflammation and other risk factors of heart disease and stroke. Furthermore, it's an extraordinary souce of protein, which is significant for managing blood sugar.

2. **Egg:**

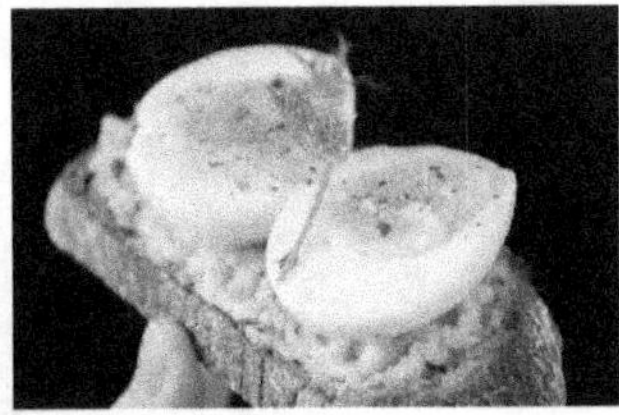

Eggs might further develop risk factors for heart disease, advance great blood sugar management, safeguard eye well-being, and keep you feeling full.

3. **Squash:**

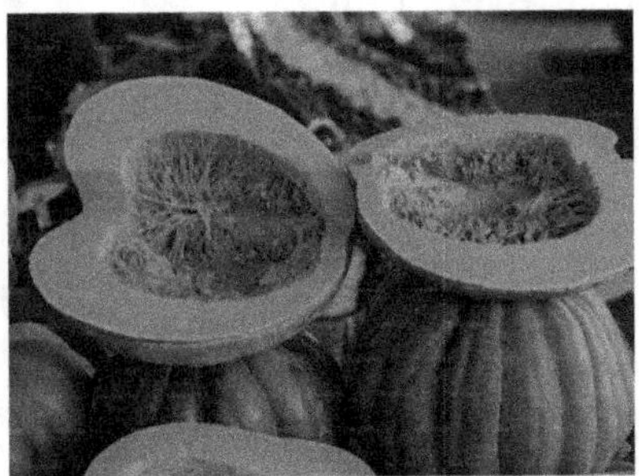

Summer and winter squash contain gainful cell reinforcements and may assist with bringing down blood sugar.

4. **Extra-virgin olive oil:**

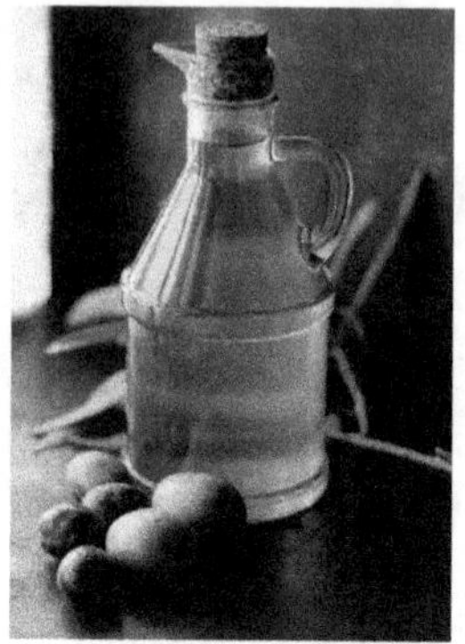

Extra-virgin olive oil contains solid oleic
corrosiveness. It has benefits for pulse and
heart wellbeing.

5. **Beans:**

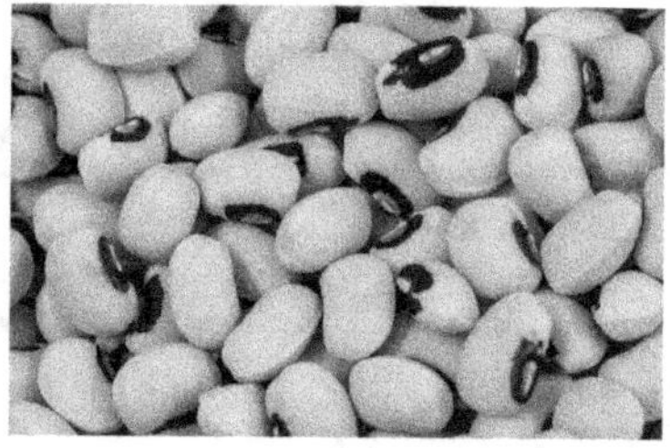

Beans are modest, nutritious, and have a low
glycemic record, making them a solid choice
for individuals with diabetes.

6. **Nuts:**

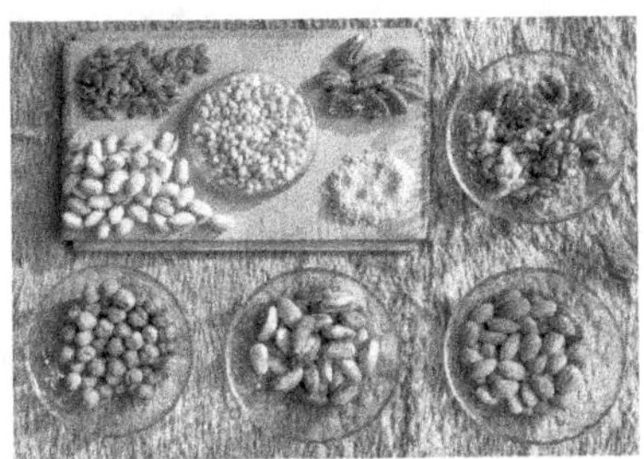

Nuts are a sound addition to a balanced diet. They're high in fiber and can assist with reducing blood sugar and LDL (Bad) cholesterol levels.

7. **Garlic:**

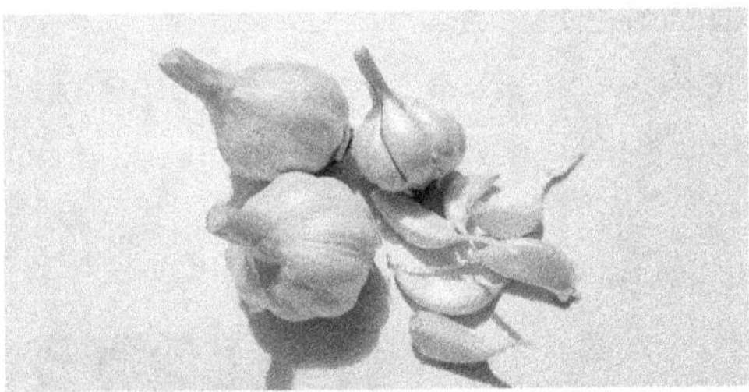

Based on research, garlic can assist with reducing blood pressure and managing cholesterol levels. Garlic assists in lowering blood sugar, irritation, LDL cholesterol, and blood pressure in individuals with diabetes.

Furthermore, specific fruits recommended for people with diabetes include:

Apple, Avocados, Guava, Blueberry, Strawberries, Cherries, Orange, Kiwi, Whole Grains like earthy brown rice, barley, oat, and Bulgur wheat.

Specific Foods to Avoid

Similarly as significant as sorting out which food sources you should include in a for diabetes is understanding which food sources you should limit. This is because numerous food sources and beverages are high in carbs and added sugar, which can cause sugar levels to spike. Different food varieties could adversely influence heart health or add to weight gain.

The following are a couple of foods that you should restrict or stay away from if you have diabetes.

1. **Alcohol**:

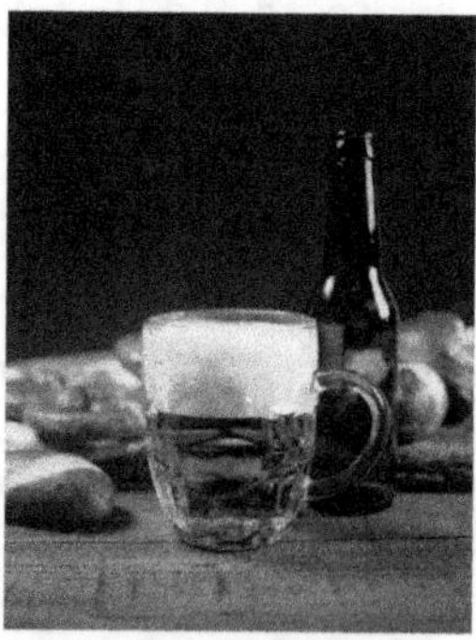

People with diabetes are by and large encouraged to restrict their alcohol consumption. This is because alcohol can increase the risk of low blood sugar, particularly whenever consumed while starving.

2. **Fried food**:

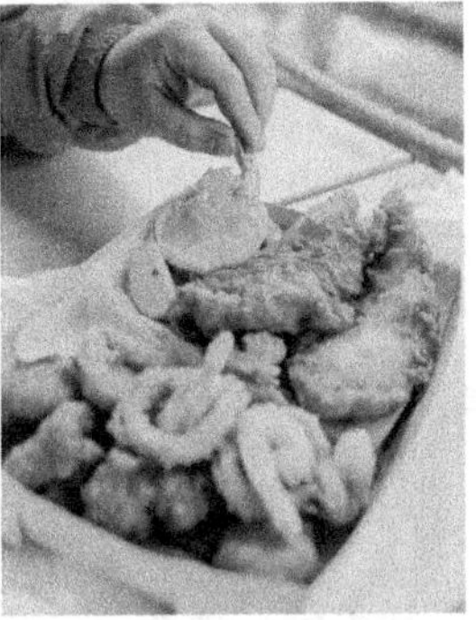

Fried food sources have a ton of trans fat, a sort of fat that has been connected to a higher risk of heart disease. In addition, fried food sources like potato chips, french fries, and mozzarella sticks are additionally normally high in calories, which could contribute to weight gain.

3. **Candy**:

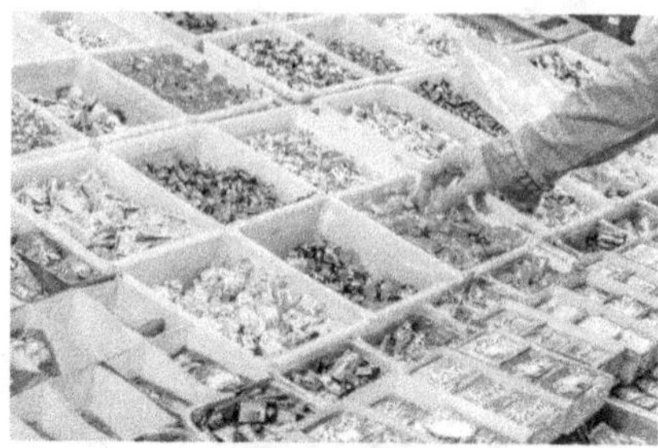

Each serving of candy contains a significant
amount of sugar. It ordinarily has a high
glycemic file, meaning it's probably going to
cause spikes and crashes in blood sugar
levels after you eat.

4. **Processed meats**:

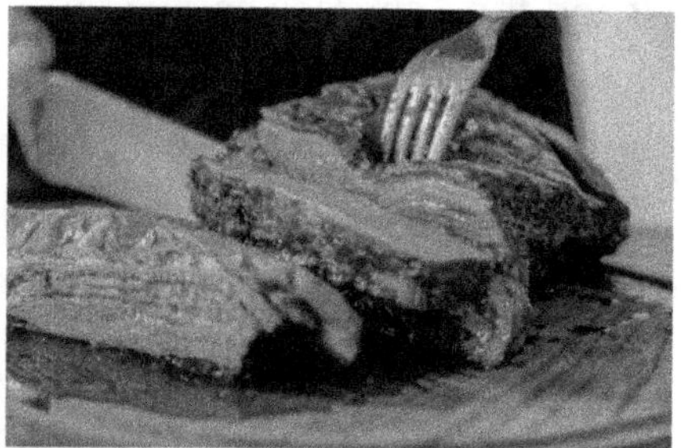

Processed meats like bacon, wieners, salami,
and cold cuts are high in sodium, additives,
and other unsafe mixtures. Besides,
processed meats have been related to a
higher risk of heart disease.

5. **Refined grains**:

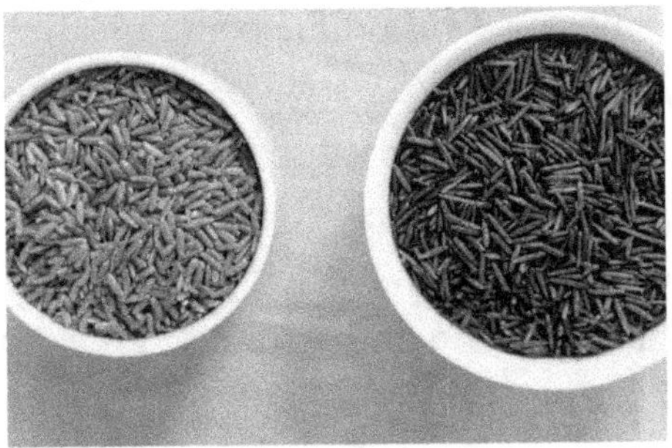

Refined grains like white bread, pasta, and rice are high in carbs, but low in fiber, which can raise blood sugar levels more rapidly than their entire grain counterparts. As indicated by research, whole-grain rice was fundamentally more effective at stabilizing blood sugar levels after eating than white rice.

6. **Fruit juice**:

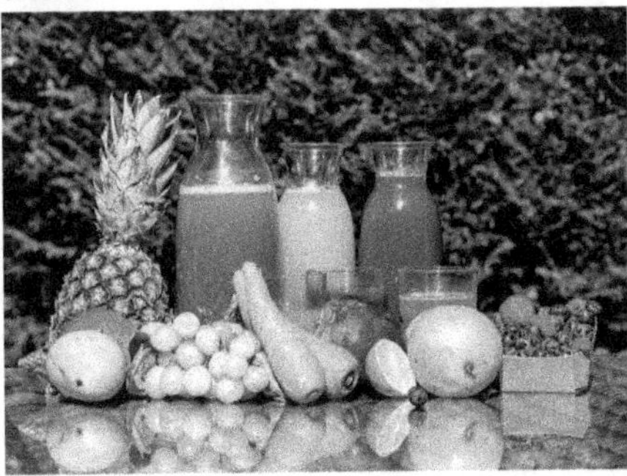

Although 100% fruit juice can be delighted now and then in moderation, it's ideal to adhere to the whole fruit whenever the situation allows if you have diabetes. This is because fruit juice contains all the carbs and sugar tracked down in fresh fruit, yet it lacks the fiber needed to assist with settling glucose levels.

Specific fruits to avoid for people with diabetes are Bananas, Watermelon, Grapes, Pineapple, Mangos, Dried organic product, Stick organic product.

Eating for Mental Well-being

Nutrition plays a crucial role in mental health. Consume foods rich in omega-3 fatty acids, such as fatty fish and walnuts, which may improve mood and cognitive function. Ensure a diverse diet with a wide range of nutrients to support overall mental well-being.

Eating for specific goals during dieting involves tailoring your food choices to align with your objectives. Whether you aim to lose weight, gain muscle, improve athletic performance, or manage specific health conditions, a balanced diet that meets your unique needs is essential. To achieve long-term results, keep in mind that consistency and patience are essential.

Chapter 6
The perfect two weeks weight loss plan

This is a comprehensive and dynamic 2-week weight loss plan designed to help you achieve your fitness goals. This thoughtfully crafted program combines balanced nutrition, invigorating exercise, and essential self-care to guide you on your journey toward a healthier and more energetic you. With a focus on nourishing meals, engaging workouts, mindful practices, and ample hydration, this plan offers a holistic approach to weight loss that promotes sustainability and well-being. Embark on this exciting adventure with dedication, enthusiasm, and the knowledge that positive changes await you over the next two weeks.

Week 1 (Day 1 to 7)
Day 1

Breakfast:

- Start your day with a warm bowl of cereal made with rolled oats and water or milk. Add a modest bunch of new berries (like blueberries, strawberries, or raspberries) for natural sweetness and antioxidants. Top with a little handful of chopped nuts (like almonds or pecans) for solid fats and added texture.

Lunch:

- craft fair, a wonderful barbecued chicken serving of mixed greens. Begin with a bed of leafy greens or spinach. Add cut barbecued chicken bosom, cherry tomatoes, cucumber cuts, ringer pepper strips, and red onion rings. Sprinkle a basic vinaigrette made with olive oil, lemon juice, Dijon mustard, and a touch of honey for some flavor.

Snack:

- For a mid-afternoon shot in the arm, enjoy a little bowl of Greek yogurt with a sprinkle of cinnamon and a couple of cucumber cuts as an afterthought. Greek yogurt's protein content keeps you feeling full.

Dinner:

- Set up a deliciously prepared fish dish. Season a fillet of your number one fish (like salmon or tilapia) with spices like dill, lemon zing, and a bit of olive oil. Roast it in the oven alongside a blend of steamed broccoli florets and a serving of cooked quinoa.

Cardio:

- To get your heart rate up and your muscles moving, require a lively 30-minute walk in your area or a close by park. This moderate cardio exercise will help start your metabolism for the day.

Water:

- focus on drinking not less than 8 glasses (64 ounces) of water throughout the day.

Sleep: Aim for 7 to 9 hours of sleep each day.

Day 2

Breakfast:

- Make a protein-pressed breakfast by scrambling eggs with diced spinach and a sprinkle of low-fat cheese. Serve the eggs on a cut of whole-grain toast for supported energy.

Lunch:

- Gather a turkey and avocado wrap. Spread out an entire grain tortilla and layer on cut turkey, rich avocado, spinach leaves, and a thin spread of Dijon mustard. Roll it up and enjoy a fair blend of protein, healthy fats, and veggies.

Snacks:

- Cut a medium apple and match it with a tablespoon of almond spread. This snack gives a delightful mix of natural sugars, fiber, and healthy fats.

Dinner:

- For a delightful and nutrient-rich dinner, stir and fry tofu cube with a variety of vivid veggies like chime peppers, snap peas, and carrots. Season with a light teriyaki or soy-ginger sauce. Serve over a portion of cooked brown rice for complex carbs.

Cardio:

- spice up your cardio routine with a 30-minute cycling session. Whether you're on an exercise bike or cycling outside, this movement helps burn calories and work on cardiovascular health.

Water:

- Aim to drink at least 8 glasses (64 ounces) of water over the day.

Rest: Ensure you get 7 to 9 hours of sleep for the day.

Day 3

Breakfast:

- Prepare a refreshing Greek yogurt parfait. Layer plain Greek yogurt with your number one granola for crunch, and afterward add a combination of diced blended natural products like strawberries, kiwi, and pineapple on top.

Lunch:

- Enjoy a soothing bowl of lentil soup. If you're in a rush, decide on a store-bought, low-sodium form. Pair it with a side plate of mixed greens made out of leafy greens, cherry tomatoes, cucumbers, and a shower of balsamic vinaigrette.

Snack:

- Snatch a handful of mixed nuts, like almonds, pecans, and cashews. These nuts give solid fats and protein to keep you satisfied.

Dinner:

- Set up a lean protein and vegetable combo by barbecuing a steak and serving it with simmered Brussels sprouts and baked sweet potato. Sprinkle the vegetables with a hint of olive oil and season with spices and herbs.

Cardio:

- Lace-up your running shoes and set out on a 30-minute run. Running is an effective method for burning calories and working on cardiovascular endurance.

Water:

- Plan to drink no less than 8 glasses (64 ounces) of water over the day.

Sleep: Go for 7 to 9 hours of sleep daily.

Day 4

Breakfast:

- Mix a nutrient-packed smoothie using a handful of spinach, one ripped banana, unsweetened almond milk, and a scoop of your number one protein powder. Add a tablespoon of chia seeds for an additional increase in fiber.

Lunch:

- Prepare a satisfying quinoa and dark bean bowl. Begin with cooked quinoa as the base, then, at that point, layer on dark beans, diced tomatoes, corn portions, diced red onion, and chopped cilantro. Shower with a squeeze of lime juice.

Snack:

- Enjoy a little bowl of curds finished off with cut peaches for a reasonable and protein-rich tidbit.

Dinner:

- Grill a salmon fillet prepared with lemon zing, garlic, and a touch of salt. Serve alongside steamed asparagus lances and a scoop of cooked wild rice.

Water:

- Aim to drink somewhere around 8 glasses (64 ounces) of water over the day.

Sleep: Ensure you get 7 to 9 hours sleep for the day.

Day 5

Breakfast:

- prepare a hearty breakfast by layering curds and cut strawberries on whole-grain toast. The mix of protein, fiber, and nutrients will assist with keeping you satisfied throughout the morning.

Lunch:

- Specialty tasty chickpea and vegetable sautéed food. Sauté chickpeas with a mix of bright vegetables like chime peppers, zucchini, and snap peas. Toss them in a light soy sauce or teriyaki sauce for added flavor.

Snack:

- Enjoy in a handful of small carrots and celery sticks with a side of hummus. This tidbit gives crunch, fiber, and a delightful plunge.

Dinner:

- Heat chicken bosom with a marinade of lemon juice, minced garlic, and a sprinkle of dried spices. Serve with broiled zucchini and a liberal part of whole grain couscous.

Cardio:

- Partak in a 30-minute stop-and-go aerobic exercise (HIIT) exercise. Shift back and forth between 30 seconds of extreme activity (like bouncing jacks, burpees, or high knees) and 30 seconds of rest.

Water:

- Aim to drink at least 8 glasses (64 ounces) of water throughout the day.

Sleep: Go for 7 to 9 hours of sleep for the day.

Day 6

Breakfast:

- Enjoy fried egg whites cooked with diced tomatoes and a touch of cleaved basil. Serve on whole-grain toast for a balanced breakfast.

Lunch:

- Make a vibrant spinach salad including barbecued shrimp as the protein source. Add crumbled feta cheddar, cherry tomatoes, and red onion cuts. Sprinkle with balsamic vinaigrette.

Snack:

- Spread almond margarine on rice cakes for a crunchy and protein-rich tidbit.

Dinner:

- prepare stuffed ringer peppers by filling split peppers with a combination of lean ground turkey, cooked brown rice, diced tomatoes, and flavors. Heat until the peppers are delicate and the filling is cooked through.

Cardio:

- Engage in a 30-minute swimming meeting. Swimming offers a full-body exercise and is delicate on the joints.

Water:

- Aim to drink something like 8 glasses (64 ounces) of water over the day.

Rest: Strive for at least 7 to 9 hours of sleep for the day

Day 7

Breakfast:

- Start your day with a bowl of overnight oats for breakfast. Blend rolled oats with chia seeds, almond milk, and a little bit of honey. Allow the mixture to be in the fridge short term. In the morning, top with a sliced banana and a sprinkle of cinnamon.

Lunch:

- Create a whole grain wrap with lean turkey cuts, lettuce, and sliced tomatoes. Spread a thin layer of hummus for added flavor and smoothness.

Snack:

- Make a mixed fruit bowl using different fresh fruits like strawberries, blueberries, grapes, and melon solid cubes.

Dinner:

- Plan barbecued vegetables and tofu sticks. Thread tofu shapes and a beautiful grouping of vegetables, (such as chime peppers, zucchini, and red onion) onto sticks. Place on top of quinoa that has been cooked.

Water:

- Aim to drink about 8 glasses (64 ounces) of water over the day.

Rest day:

- Allow your body to recover and re-energize. Rest days are important for muscle fixing and general well-being. Go for at least 7 hours of sleep.

Week 2 (Day 8 to 14)

Go on with the balanced diet and snacks from Week 1

Day 8

Try a new exercise class or routine to keep things energizing. Exploring different exercises forestalls boredom as well as challenges your body in new ways. Whether it's a dance exercise, a high-intensity exercise class, or an outdoor training camp, variety can be effective and motivating.

Water: Aim to drink 8 glasses (64 ounces) of water over the day.

Sleep: Aim for 7-9 hours of sleep.

Day 9

During your training session, focus on increasing the weight or opposition for certain exercises. For instance, if you were using 5-pound hand weights for bicep twists, have a go at using 7.5-pound hand weights. This dynamic overload helps stimulate muscle development and strength development.

Water: Intend to drink somewhere around 8 glasses (64 ounces) of water over the day.

Sleep: Get a quality sleep of 7 to 9 hours for the day.

Day 10

Practise mindful eating during your dinners. Set aside distractions like phones and televisions, and eat slowly. Focus on the taste, texture, and satisfaction of each bite. This careful methodology can assist you in enjoying your food more and perceiving when you're comfortably full.

Day 11

During your cardio session, consider integrating intervals. Shift back and forth between times of higher power and times of lower force. For instance, alternate between a 2-minute jog and a 1-minute jog for a sum of 20-30 minutes.

Day 12

Try different things with another healthy recipe. For dinner, think about making an enormous, colorful salad with different veggies, lean protein (like barbecued chicken or chickpeas), and a homemade constructed vinaigrette dressing. A vibrant salad can be both satisfying and nutritious.

Day 13

Devote time to relaxation techniques like profound breathing, meditation, or yoga. Search for a quiet area, settle in, and focus on your breathing. Deep breathing and mindfulness exercises can assist in reducing pressure and promote mental clarity.

Day 14

Reflect on your progress throughout the past two weeks. Take a moment to acknowledge any positive changes you've experienced, whether it's increased energy, further developed fitness, or a feeling of achievement. Use this reflection to set a new goal and adjust your plan on a case-by-case basis.

Strength training: Take part in a full-body strength instructional meeting. Start with a warm-up that includes dynamic stretches and portability works out. For your workouts, focus on compound developments, such as squats, jumps, push-ups, planks, and rows. Go for three sets of 10-12 reps for each exercise.

Remember that the weight loss journey is remarkable for everybody. Adjust the plan to suit your preferences and lifestyle. Consistency, persistence, and a positive mindset are essential for accomplishing and keeping up with your weight loss goals.

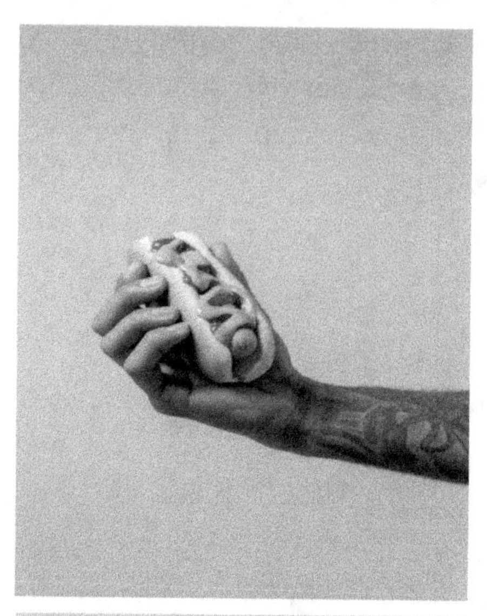

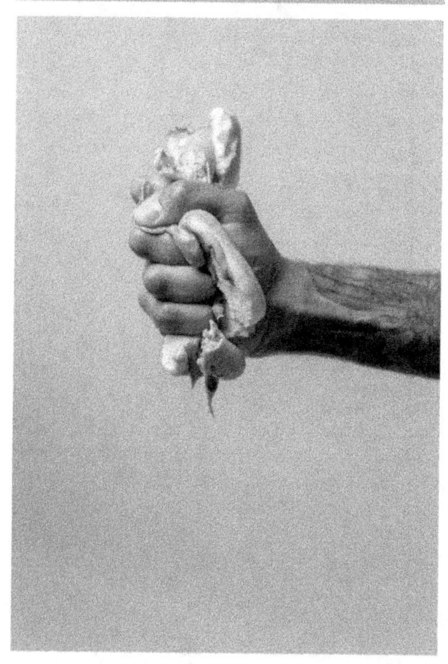

Chapter 7

The Anti-inflammatory diet

Before delving into anti-inflammatories, you need to know what inflammation is.

Inflammation is when your body protects itself from disease, contamination, or injury. Inflammation is a characteristic of a natural process that helps your body heal and defend itself from harm. As a component of the inflammatory response, your body increases its production of white blood cells, immune cells, and substances called cytokines that assist in fighting disease. Exemplary signs of acute (short-term) inflammation include redness, pain, swelling, and heat.

An anti-inflammatory diet is generally regarded as healthy. If you have a condition like rheumatoid joint inflammation, changing what's on your plate won't be a cure. However, eating less food that is inflammatory may help you experience fewer eruptions or experience less pain overall. Regardless of whether it assists with your condition, it can assist with bringing down your possibility of having other problems. If you have a condition that causes Inflammation, it might assist with changing your eating patterns.

On the other hand, inflammation is dangerous if it becomes chronic.

Chronic (long-term) inflammation frequently occurs inside your body with no observable side effects. Chronic inflammation may last for weeks, months, or years and may prompt different health problems. This kind of inflammation has been linked to diseases like cancer, fatty liver disease, diabetes, and heart disease. Chronic inflammation can likewise happen when people are obese or under pressure. At the point when specialists search for information, they test for a couple of markers in your blood, including C-responsive protein (CRP), homocysteine, TNF alpha, and IL-6. Inflammation is a defensive mechanism that allows your body to protect itself against disease, sickness, or injury. It can likewise occur on a chronic basis, which can lead to various diseases.

What Causes inflammation

Certain lifestyle factors, particularly habitual ones, can promote Inflammation. High fructose corn syrup and sugar consumption is particularly harmful. It can lead to insulin obstruction, diabetes, and weight Researchers have likewise guessed that consuming a ton of refined carbs, like white bread, may contribute to inflammation, insulin resistance, and obesity. Eating processed and bundled food varieties that contain trans fats has been viewed to promote Inflammation and harm the endothelial cells that line your arteries. The FDA has considered trans fats no more "Generally recognized as safe," so most food should no longer have trans fats. Vegetable oils used in many processed food sources are another possible culprit. Regular Consumption may result in an imbalance of omega-6 to omega-3 unsaturated fats, which some researchers believe may promote Inflammation. Excess consumption of alcohol and processed meat can also have an inflammatory effect on your body. Moreover, an inactive lifestyle that includes a lot of sitting is a significant non-dietary factor that promotes Inflammation. Eating unhealthy food, drinking alcohol or sweet refreshments, and getting little physical activity are undeniably associated with increased inflammation.

The role and impact of Your diet

If you want to reduce Inflammation, eat less inflammatory food sources and more anti-inflammatory food. Base your diet on whole, nutrient-dense food that contains antioxidants, and stay away from highly processed products with lots of added sugar and oils. Antioxidants work by reducing degrees of free radicals. These responsive molecules are made as a natural part of your metabolism but can lead to inflammation when they're not kept in check. Your anti-inflammatory diet should provide a healthy balance of protein, carbs, and fat at every meal. Ensure you likewise meet your body's needs for nutrients, minerals, fiber, and water.

One diet considered anti-inflammatory is the Mediterranean diet, which has been shown to decrease inflammatory markers, like CRP and IL-6. A low-carb diet likewise reduces Inflammation, especially for people with obesity or metabolic conditions. Furthermore, vegetarian diets are linked to reducing Inflammation. Choose a nutrient-dense diet that removes processed foods and increases your intake of whole, inflammatory- and antioxidant-rich foods.

5 of the Most Anti-inflammatory Food Sources You Can Eat

1. Fruits and Vegetables: Fruits and vegetables are rich in vitamins, minerals, and antioxidants that combat inflammation. Berries, such as blueberries, contain anthocyanins that help reduce oxidative stress and inflammation. Leafy greens like spinach and kale provide a high dose of vitamin K, which supports bone health and has anti-inflammatory effects. These greens are also rich in fiber, which supports a healthy gut microbiome.

2. Fatty Fish: Fatty fish, including salmon, mackerel, sardines, and trout, are brimming with long-chain omega-3 fatty acids like EPA and DHA. These omega-3s are essential for reducing inflammation at the cellular level, promoting heart health, and supporting brain function.

3. Nuts and Seeds: Nuts and seeds have lots of nutrients, and many anti-inflammatory foods like vitamin E and ellagitannins (a type of tannin). Walnuts are unique among nuts because they are high in ALA, a plant-based omega-3 fatty acid. Flaxseeds and chia seeds provide both omega-3s and fiber, supporting heart health and reducing inflammation. Nuts and seeds are also a source of healthy fats that help with nutrient absorption and provide satiety. Nuts include Almonds, cashews, chestnuts, hazelnuts, pine nuts, pistachios, and pecans. Seeds include Pumpkin seeds, sunflower seeds, and sesame seeds.

4. Whole Grains: Whole grains like brown rice, quinoa, and whole wheat contain complex carbohydrates and fiber. Fiber helps maintain stable blood sugar levels, reduces inflammation, and supports gut health by nourishing beneficial gut bacteria. Additionally, whole grains provide an array

of vitamins and minerals. More examples of whole grains are Barley, BuckwheatBrown, Oats, Sorghum (a grain well known in parts of Asia and Africa), Whole rye, and Whole wheat (bulgur wheat and wheat berries).

5. Healthy Fats: Olive oil or extra virgin oil is rich in monounsaturated fats and contains antioxidants that fight inflammation and oxidative stress. Avocados are another source of monounsaturated fats and are packed with potassium, which helps regulate blood pressure.

6. Spices and Herbs: Turmeric contains curcumin, a potent anti-inflammatory compound that has been studied for its potential to reduce inflammation and alleviate symptoms of chronic conditions. Ginger has gingerol, an anti-inflammatory compound that can help ease nausea and muscle pain. Garlic contains allicin, known for its potential to lower inflammation and support heart health. Cinnamon has been linked to improved insulin sensitivity and reduced inflammation.

7. Green Tea: Green tea contains catechins, powerful antioxidants that have been shown to reduce inflammation and support cellular health. Drinking green tea regularly is associated with a decreased risk of chronic

diseases and may aid in weight management.

8. Probiotic-Rich Foods: Probiotic-rich foods like yogurt, kefir, sauerkraut, and kimchi contain live beneficial bacteria that promote a healthy gut microbiome. A healthy gut microbiome has been linked to lowered inflammation and enhanced immune performance.

The few food sources that are associated with an increased risk of chronic inflammation.

The specific Foods to Avoid include:

1. Processed Foods: Highly processed foods often contain refined sugars, unhealthy fats, and additives that contribute to inflammation. These foods lack the nutrients needed for a healthy body and can lead to weight gain, insulin resistance, and chronic diseases.

2. Refined Carbohydrates: Refined carbohydrates, such as white bread and sugary cereals, are quickly absorbed by the body and cause rapid spikes in blood sugar levels. This can trigger an inflammatory response and contribute to metabolic disorders.

3. Sugary Beverages: Sugar-sweetened beverages are major sources of added

sugars, which can promote inflammation, weight gain, and insulin resistance. Consider drinking water, herbal teas, or unsweetened alternatives instead.

4. Red and Processed Meats: Red meats like beef, pork, and lamb, as well as processed meats like sausages and bacon, contain saturated fats and potentially harmful compounds. High consumption has been linked to inflammation, cardiovascular disease, and certain cancers.

5. Highly Saturated Fats: Foods high in saturated fats, including full-fat dairy products and fatty cuts of meat, can contribute to chronic inflammation and increase the risk of heart disease. Choose lean protein sources and lower-fat dairy options.

6. Excessive Alcohol: Alcohol consumption, especially in excess, can lead to inflammation and oxidative stress in various organs, including the liver. Moderation is key to minimizing the negative effects of inflammation.

7. Trans Fats: Trans fats are artificially created fats found in some fried and processed foods. They increase inflammation, raise bad cholesterol levels, and contribute to

heart disease. Always check food labels to avoid trans fats.

A One-Day sample Menu you can use

It's simpler to adhere to a diet when you have an arrangement or plan. Here is a great sample menu to begin you out, highlighting a day of anti-inflammatory meals.

Breakfast

- a three-egg omelet cooked in olive oil with a cup (110 grams) of mushrooms and a cup (67 grams) of kale1 cup (225 grams) of cherries.
- Green tea as well as water.

Lunch

- Barbecued salmon on a bed of leafy greens with olive oil and vinegar
- 1 cup (125 grams) of raspberries, topped with plain Greek yogurt and cleaved walnuts
- Unsweetened chilled tea, water.

Snack

- Bell pepper strips with guacamole.

Dinner

- Chicken curry with sweet potato, cauliflower, and broccoli
- Red wine (5-10 ounces or 140-280 ml)

- 1 ounce (30 grams) of dark chocolate (ideally no less than 80% cocoa).

An anti-inflammatory diet plan should be well-balanced, including food with helpful impacts at each dinner.

Other beneficial supplements

When you have your healthy menu coordinated, ensure you integrate these other beneficial routines of an anti-inflammatory lifestyle:

- Supplements: Fish oil and curcumin are two supplements that have been shown to reduce inflammation.
- Regular exercise: Exercise can reduce inflammatory markers and your risk of chronic disease.
- Sleep: Getting enough sleep is crucial. Poor sleep, according to research, makes inflammation worse..

You can boost the advantages of your anti-inflammatory diet by taking supplements and making sure to get sufficient exercise and sleep.

Benefits of anti-inflammatory diet

An inflammatory diet, alongside exercise and good sleep, may provide many advantages:

Improvement of symptoms of joint pain, inflammatory bowel disease, lupus, and other immune system problems

Decreasing the risk of obesity, heart disease, diabetes, depression, cancer, and other diseases.

Decrease in inflammatory markers in your blood.

Better blood sugar, cholesterol, and fatty oil levels.

Improvement in energy and state of mind.

Following an anti-inflammatory diet and way of life might further develop markers of Inflammation and reduce your risk of numerous diseases. Chronic Inflammation is unhealthy and can prompt illness. In many cases, your diet and lifestyle either cause or aggravate inflammation. You should aim to choose anti-inflammatory foods for ideal well-being and health, bringing down your risk of diseases.

The Dash diet

If you have been exploring various diets lately, you might have coincidentally found the Dash diet and found yourself curious about what it involves. First introduced in 1997, the Dash diet means 'dietary approach to stop hypertension' (otherwise called High blood pressure). High blood pressure affects almost 50% of all Americans and is defined as a systolic blood pressure more prominent than 130 mmHg or a diastolic blood pressure greater than 80 mmHg. High blood pressure can cause harm to a range of organs throughout the body and may result in cardiovascular failure or stroke when left untreated. The good news is, that the Dash diet offers an incredible nutrition-based method for reducing high blood pressure without you needing to roll out any sensational change to the food you're consuming. Focusing on reducing the amount of sodium consumed by encouraging people to eat whole foods.

The Dash diet emphasizes reducing red meat and highly processed food items that are high in salt and sugar while increasing potassium, magnesium, and calcium intake. Potassium, magnesium, and calcium are immensely important minerals in the regulation of blood pressure, as they take part in the relaxation and contraction of blood vessels. Likewise, potassium purging affects the sodium in the body, so the more potassium you eat, the more sodium you lose through urine.

The Dash diet explicitly meets the sodium requirement that can give people an edge over hypertension. This means it's an extraordinary diet for people who have hypertension or are looking to reduce their risk of heart disease, as well as those people who might be at risk of type 2 diabetes or are currently dealing with the condition.

DASH Diet Types

Depending on your health needs, you can select from two forms of the Dash diet.

1. The standard Dash diet This plan limits sodium consumption to 2,300 milligrams (mg) per day.
1. The lower-sodium Dash diet This type calls for limiting sodium consumption to 1,500 mg each day.

How Does the Dash Diet Lower Blood Pressure?

The Dash diet works by limiting sodium as well as Saturated fat, both of which can be hindering heart health. A diet that is heavy in salt can drive up blood pressure, which overwhelms the heart muscle. However, saturated fat can raise cholesterol levels. "Cholesterol has the potential of blocking or decreasing the flow of blood to the heart," restricted bloodstream can result in heart attack and stroke.

The effective 7 Days sample of Dash diet Menu You Can Follow

The Dash diet calls for lots of new veggies and fruits but requires just a moderate amount of whole grains, as well as a lean source of protein and healthy fats, like those from fish and nuts, respectively. This sets the Dash diet apart from other well-known programs like the Atkins diet, the ketogenic diet, and the high-fat, low-carbohydrate diet. Here is a simple seven-day meal on the Dash diet.

Day 1

Breakfast

- 1 whole wheat bagel with two tablespoons (tbsp) of unsalted peanut butter
- 1 medium orange
- 1 cup sans-fat milk
- Decaffeinated espresso.

Lunch

- Spinach salad made with 4 cups of new spinach leaves, 1 cut pear, ½ cup canned mandarin orange areas, a cup of slivered almonds, and 2 tbsp red wine vinaigrette
- 12 reduced-sodium wheat wafers
- 1 cup fat-free milk.

Snack

- 1 cup fat-free, low-calorie yogurt
- 4 vanilla wafers.

Dinner

- 3 ounces (oz) spice-crusted baked cod
- ½ cup brown rice pilaf with vegetables
- ½ cup steamed green beans
- 2 teaspoons (tsp) of olive oil and 1 small sourdough roll
- 1 cup fresh berries with slashed mint
- Herbal chilled tea.

Day 2

Breakfast

- 1 cup fresh mixed fruits finished off with 1 cup sans fat, low-calorie vanilla-seasoned yogurt, and cup walnut
- 1-grain biscuit with 1 tsp trans fat,-free margarine
- 1 cup fat-free milk
- Herbal tea.

Lunch

- Whole wheat tortilla, 1 cup chopped chicken, 1/2 cup diced apple, 1 12 tbsp light mayonnaise, and 1/2 tsp curry powder are used to make the curried chicken wrap.½ cup raw baby carrots

- 1 cup fat-free milk.

Snack

- Trail mix made with ¼ cup raisins, around 22 unsalted smaller than mini twist pretzels, and 2 tbsp sunflower seeds.

Dinner

- 1 cup cooked whole wheat spaghetti with 1 cup marinara sauce, no additional salt
- 2 cups mixed salad greens topped with 1 tbsp low-fat Caesar dressing
- 1 teaspoon of olive oil and 1 small whole wheat roll
- 1 nectarine
- Sparkling water

Day 3

Breakfast

- ¾ cup bran flakes grain with 1 cup low-fat milk
- 1 medium banana
- 1 cup whole wheat bread with 1 tsp trans-fat-free margarine
- 1 cup orange juice.

Lunch

- Fish salad made with ½ cup drained, unsalted water-packed tuna, 2 tbsp light mayonnaise, 15 grapes, and ¼ cup diced celery served on top of 2½ cups romaine lettuce
- 8 Melba toast crackers
- 1 cup without fat milk.

Snack

- 1 cup light yogurt
- 1 medium peach.

Dinner

- Using 3 oz of beef and 1 cup each of peppers, onions, mushrooms, and cherry tomatoes, create a beef and vegetable kebab.
- 1 cup cooked wild rice
- 1 cup pineapple pieces
- 4 ounces of cran-raspberry juice combined with 4 to 8 ounces of sparkling water to make a spritzer of cranberries.

Day 4

Breakfast

- 1 cup cereal topped with 1 tsp cinnamon
- 1 sliced entire wheat toast with 1 tsp trans sans fat margarine
- 1 banana

- 1 cup without fat milk.

Lunch
- ¾ cup chicken salad with 2 cuts whole wheat bread and 1 tbsp Dijon mustard
- Salad with ½ cup cucumber cuts, ½ cup tomato wedges, 1 tbsp sunflower seeds, and 1 tsp low-calorie Italian dressing
- ½ cup fruit cocktail, juice pack.

Snack
- 1 cup unsalted almonds
- ¼ cup raisins
- ½ cup without fat, no sugar added fruit yogurt.

Dinner
- 3 oz roasted beef with 2 tbsp fat-free beef sauce
- 1 cup of green beans cooked in 1/2 teaspoon of canola oil
- 1 little baked potato with 1 tbsp fat-free sharp cream, 1 tbsp decreased fat cheddar, and 1 tbsp chopped scallions
- 1 small apple
- 1 cup low-fat milk.

Day 5

Breakfast

- ½ cup instant oats
- 1 mini whole wheat bagel with 1 tbsp peanut butter
- 1 medium banana
- 1 cup low-fat milk.

Lunch

- Chicken bosom sandwich with 3 oz of skinless chicken bosom, 2 cuts whole wheat bread, 1 cut decreased fat cheddar, 1 large leaf of romaine lettuce, 2 tomato cuts, and 1 tbsp low-fat mayo
- 1 cup melon
- 1 cup squeezed apple.

Snack

- 1 cup unsalted almonds
- ¼ cup dried apricots
- 1 cup sans fat, no sugar added organic product yogurt.

Dinner

- 1 cup spaghetti with ¾ cup vegan spaghetti sauce and 3 tbsp Parmesan cheddar
- Spinach salad with 1 cup fresh spinach leaves, ¼ cup ground carrots, ¼ cup sliced mushrooms, and 1 tbsp vinaigrette dressing

- ½ cup corn (cooked from frozen)
- ½ cup canned pears, juice pack

Day 6

Breakfast

- 1 cup whole wheat bread with 1 tsp margarine
- 1 cup fat-free, no-sugar-added fruit yogurt
- 1 medium peach
- ½ cup grape juice.

Lunch

- Ham and cheddar sandwich with 2 oz low-fat, low-sodium ham, 2 slices entire wheat bread, 1 enormous leaf of romaine lettuce, 2 cuts tomato, 1 cut reduced fat cheddar, and 1 tbsp low-fat mayonnaise
- 1 cup carrot sticks.

Snack

- 2 cup unsalted almonds
- ¼ cup dried apricots
- 1 cup low-fat milk
- 1 cup apple juice.

Dinner

- Chicken and Spanish rice
- 1 teaspoon of olive oil and 1 small whole wheat roll

- 1 cup melon
- 1 cup low-fat milk.

Day 7

Breakfast
- 1 low-fat granola bar
- 1 medium banana
- ½ cup fat-free, no-sugar-added fruit yogurt
- 1 cup squeezed orange
- 1 cup low-fat milk.

Lunch
- Turkey breast sandwich with 3 oz cooked turkey, 2 cuts whole wheat bread, 1 large leaf romaine lettuce, 2 slices tomato, 2 tsp low-fat mayonnaise, and 1 tbsp Dijon mustard
- 1 cup steamed broccoli (cooked from frozen)
- 1 medium orange.

Snack
- 2 tbsp unsalted peanuts
- 1 cup low-fat milk
- ¼ cup dried apricots.

Dinner
- 3 oz prepared fish
- 1 cup scallion rice

- Spinach sauté with ½ frozen spinach, 2 tsp canola oil, and 1 tbsp fragmented, unsalted almonds.
- 1 cup carrots (cooked from frozen)
- 1 little whole wheat roll with 1 tsp margarine
- 1 small cookie.

The Dash diet is recommended for people who need to bring down blood pressure but at the same time a great choice for anybody who needs to take on a healthy diet. Because it underlines whole food sources that are naturally low in unhealthy fats and added sugars, as well as moderate portions, it might likewise lead to weight loss, the same way it did in a group of people who had non-alcoholic fatty liver disease.

Conclusion

Eat to Beat is Your Dieting Cookbook offers a compelling and well-researched perspective on achieving and maintaining a healthier lifestyle through mindful eating. Throughout the book, readers have been provided with a plethora of delicious recipes, each carefully designed to promote not only weight loss but also overall well-being. By emphasizing the importance of balanced nutrition and a varied diet, the cookbook challenges traditional dieting notions and encourages a more sustainable approach to food.

The book's exploration of the connection between different foods and their impact on metabolism, energy levels, and digestion provides readers with valuable insights into making informed dietary choices. Moreover, the inclusion of educational sections on essential nutrients, portion control, and the role of mindfulness in eating further enhances the book's practical value.

"Eat to Beat your Dieting" not only equips readers with culinary tools but also empowers them to make lasting lifestyle changes. By offering a diverse array of recipes, from quick and easy meals to more elaborate dishes, the cookbook caters to various tastes and preferences. The emphasis on using whole, unprocessed ingredients promotes a positive relationship with food and encourages readers to view cooking as an enjoyable and creative endeavor.

Ultimately, "Eat to Beat Your Dieting Cookbook", presents a holistic approach to nutrition that extends beyond calorie counting and restrictive dieting. It underscores the importance of embracing food as a source of nourishment and pleasure while simultaneously achieving health goals. Through its comprehensive content and practical advice, the book becomes a valuable companion for those seeking a more balanced, sustainable, and fulfilling way of eating.